Culture, the Status of Women, and Demographic Behaviour

Culture, the Status of Women, and Demographic Behaviour

Illustrated with the Case of India

ALAKA MALWADE BASU

CLARENDON PRESS · OXFORD
1992

Oxford University Press, Walton Street, Oxford OX2 6DP
Oxford New York Toronto
Delhi Bombay Calcutta Madras Karachi
Petaling Jaya Singapore Hong Kong Tokyo
Nairobi Dar es Salaam Cape Town
Melbourne Auckland
and associated companies in
Berlin Ibadan

Oxford is a trade mark of Oxford University Press

Published in the United States
by Oxford University Press, New York

British Library Cataloguing in Publicaton Data
Data available

Library of Congress Cataloging-in-Publication Data
Basu, Alaka M.
Culture, the status of women, and demographic behaviour/Alaka M Basu.
p.   cm.
Includes bibliographical references (p.   ) and index.
1. Fertility, Human—India—Delhi.   2. Mortality—India—Delhi.
3. Rural-urban migration—India—Delhi.   4. Women—India—Delhi.
I. Title.
HB1050.D45B38   1992   305.4′0954′56—dc20   91–36547
ISBN 0–19–828360–1

Typeset by Spantech Publishers Pvt Ltd, New Delhi 110060
Printed and bound in Great Britain by
Biddles Ltd, Guildford and King's Lynn

To My Parents

Preface and Acknowledgements

THE work on this book began simply enough. All I originally intended to do was to test in the field some hypotheses about the effects of maternal characteristics on demographic behaviour in general and childhood mortality in particular. The usual method would have been to do some kind of retrospective survey of ever-married or currently married women, in which information was collected on a range of fairly standard socio-economic variables and a range of demographic variables, the primary ones being the numbers of children ever born and the numbers alive at the time of the survey. But the literature swarmed with the analyses of such data-sets, especially after the results from the World Fertility Survey became available, many such analyses exhibiting a technical sophistication outside the reach of a non-statistician interested in demography. At the other end of the scale were the scores of fascinating ethnographic and anthropological studies, which, however, were often localized to the point of being unique, relied entirely on description with no attempt at quantification, and, though they probed motivations and mechanisms, had only a tangential interest in demographic behaviour as a significant outcome variable.

Three independent but relatively simultaneous developments changed the course of this study. First, there was the sudden and swift appropriation by demographic research of the methods of statistics and of anthropology in a single investigation, so that quantitative estimates were enriched with qualitative insights. Secondly, we gained access to the provocative findings from several painstaking studies in historical demography, notable among these being the Princeton European Fertility Project. These studies highlighted the role of non-economic factors in explaining fertility differentials and change, such non-economic factors being encompassed in general categories such as 'culture' and 'region'. Thirdly, I discovered that the slums of Delhi provide an almost laboratory setting for doing cross-cultural studies that are uncontaminated by the effects of cross-cultural differences in the physical environment or in the environment of opportunities and services available. In some of these large slums, migrants from a range of socio-cultural and regional backgrounds live rubbing shoulders and, in spite of the common thread of poverty that runs through their lives, behave visibly differently from each other and respond visibly differently to the common extra-domestic influences on their lives.

These three developments brought together in my mind several seemingly unconnected concepts—women's status, culture, fertility, and mortality; sex differentials in mortality and well-being; the proximate determinants of fertility and mortality; behavioural mechanisms; a controlled environment. It was not long before these fell into a pattern and led naturally to ideas for a field project on the relations between cultural background and the status of women on the one hand, and the status of women and demographic behaviour on the other, the environment being controlled not statistically during data analysis but actually at the stage of data collection itself.

Within this general framework, the present study has attempted to display three distinguishing features. First, it has tried to understand a range of demographic parameters in terms of culture and women's status. Most similar studies have tended to focus on fertility and concentrate on the desire and need for children in different cultural contexts. Here, the data also allow one to look at the relations between women's status and their child mortality experience as well as gender differences in well-being; the latter have a particularly sharp relationship to women's status and roles. Secondly, there is an emphasis on the behavioural mechanisms which mediate these relationships. How does the position of women affect child mortality, for example? Does it operate through better health behaviour within the home? Or through unintentional bio-demographic factors? Or is it simply a result of having more money? Such detailed interpretations were more possible because, in addition to the retrospective survey, there was a six-month period of longitudinal data collection and observation which gave as much importance to garnering qualitative information as to the accumulation of quantifiable data on behaviour. And thirdly, this study has tried to examine the applicability of our knowledge based on the experience of the developed world to the present situation in a typical developing country.

But field research is a costly business. There are questionnaires to be printed, weighing machines to be bought, field investigators to be employed. For making all this possible, I would like to thank Sheila Macrae and the Overseas Development Administration, London, for a generous grant (no. R3934) to the National Council of Applied Economic Research, New Delhi, for the project. I also appreciate their forbearance when the final study report was not forthcoming by the appointed date.

Being a somewhat itinerant employee, I have to thank several different places of work for their faculty, their libraries, and their research facilities. I shall mention three in particular. First, there is the National Council of Applied Economic Research in New Delhi, where I was based during the fieldwork and the initial primary data analysis; this institution provided the kind of support for field research that other places can often only dream of. Then there is the Office of Population Research at Princeton University, where I was a Visiting Fellow during the period 1989–90 and where the manuscript proceeded handsomely thanks to the office's lively work and interpersonal environment. Finally, my gratitude to the Institute of Economic Growth, Delhi, where I am currently based, the faculty of which includes several non-demographers with a healthy interest in demography, ever ready to offer a willing ear either during a seminar or over tea.

As for individuals, my list is long and often daunting in its luminary content. The latter is a testimonial not to my special qualities, but to the extraordinary inability to say no among those that haunt the corridors of power in demographic research. My first and perhaps largest debt is to my teacher and guide William Brass. While I think he is still unsure whether this is the kind of demographic research he trained me for, I, for my part, have to hold him primarily responsible for my interest in population studies and for my switch from the biological to the social sciences. Quite apart from his teaching, I think Professor Brass needs to be singled out for the weight of his encouragement, friendliness, and humour, all of which his former students can gratefully testify to.

Then, there are those who worked with me, commented on my writings, or stimulated me with their discussions. In alphabetical order, those I would like to thank in particular are: Peter Aaby, Sajeda Amin, Kaushik Basu, Usha Basu, Idrak Bhatty, Ashish

Bose, Gitarani Bhowmik, John Caldwell, Pat Caldwell, Lincoln Chen, John Cleland, Ansley Coale, Nigel Crook, Tim Dyson, Jhiki Ganguli, Cynthia Lloyd, Carolyn Makinson, Indu Malwade, Ramesh Malwade, Moni Nag, Amartya Sen, D. V. Sethi, John Simons, Ramamani Sundar, James Trussell, and Leela Visaria. However, much as I would like to hide behind some of these illustrious names, I admit that all errors, misinterpretations and plain stupidities are my responsibility entirely.

The field-workers, especially the women, deserve a special mention as the quantitative as well as qualitative data would have been infinitely poorer without their insights, enthusiasm, and resilience, especially during the collection of longitudinal data, which continued through a scorching June and a slushy August. Accordingly, I place on record my gratitude to Madhu Mittal, Narinder Kaur, Vijay Thapliyal, Charulekha, Kusumlata, Sunita Saini, Chitra Ganapaty, Vimala Srinivasan, Vijayalakshmi Moorthy, Anuradha Seshadri, and K. Subhalakshmi.

It is customary to end one's acknowledgements with a special word for the 'understanding support' of one's family. While I think Kaushik deserves mention, especially for his impatience with logically loose statements, I am inclined otherwise to plagiarize P. G. Wodehouse and thank him, Karna, and Diksha as well as my sisters Anuradha, Anjali, and Amita, 'without whose never failing sympathy and encouragement this book would have been finished in half the time' (Wodehouse, 1926).

Institute of Economic Growth, Delhi   Alaka Basu

Contents

Figures

Tables

1

Introduction

THAT demographic behaviour is not purely, and some would say not even primarily, a function of immediate economic factors has been a view in the demographic literature for some time now. This view has received considerable support from two independent lines of inquiry, one concerned with the processes of historical fertility declines and the other focusing on cross-sectional differences in fertility and in infant and child mortality in contemporary populations.[1] In both these cases, it quickly became apparent that explanations based on economic causes could go only so far. There remained a hard core of observations that required explanations which, for want of a better expression, one may refer to as extra-economic.

The present study is an attempt to identify some of these extra-economic influences on demographic behaviour. It begins by recognizing that region or culture is an important correlate of demographic behaviour. Next, it tries to identify the attributes of a region or culture which might be the actual determinant of such behaviour and concludes that, in the Indian case at least, and possibly in several other areas with cultural differences in demographic indicators, the status of women is a prominent determining attribute. The study then tries to make a more general argument in favour of a significant connection between the status of women, as defined in specific ways, and demographic behaviour, as measured by fertility, child mortality, and gender differences in physical welfare. A predominant feature is the attempt to identify the proximate determinants in the observed connections between women's roles and these measures of demographic behaviour.

While the main objective of this book is to make a general case for a systematic relationship between culture or region and women's status on the one hand, and between women's status and demographic behaviour on the other, the Indian evidence is used to illustrate such a case. Hence, the bulk of the empirical support for the study comes from a comparison of two distinct regional groups in India, one North Indian and the other South Indian. And the bulk of this North-South analysis is based on primary data collected from a multicultural slum in the city of Delhi. Two groups of first-generation migrants were selected, one set belonging to two contiguous districts in the eastern part of the state of Uttar Pradesh (to represent the largely Hindi-speaking northern part of the country), and the other set belonging to four contiguous districts in Tamil Nadu (to represent the culturally distinct southern part of the country).[2] Since both groups belonged to the lowest rungs of the socio-economic ladder, the study was able to control to a large extent for socio-economic status as a determinant of demographic behaviour (in any case, most analyses take the small socio-economic differentials into account). At the same time, by choosing these two cultural groups living in the same area, one got almost a laboratory situation as far as the external physical environment as well as the theoretical access to services and opportunities were concerned.

As argued later in the book, there is little evidence that the two sets of migrants were a specially selected group with reference to their region of origin or with reference to each other, but in subsequent chapters an attempt is nevertheless made to back up the field findings with secondary data from the two states of origin (the rural areas, as these are more homogeneous than the aggregate urban areas as a whole). In recent years there has been a spate of fairly detailed data analyses available from the census as well as several large-scale (usually government-sponsored) surveys, and I therefore try to use the published results of these data analyses, in addition to the primary data collected during the field survey, to throw some light on the mechanisms involved in the observed links between culture and demographic behaviour, and the role of socio-economic differentials in obscuring or heightening this link. Of necessity, the kinds of links explored involve much use of non-quantitative data, especially for the independent variables, but wherever possible an effort is made to relate these to outcome measures which can be quantified.

To explain the regional differential in demographic variables in terms of cultural practices and norms, one needs first to remove socio-economic factors as a confounding variable. In the present study, this is done by focusing on groups that fall within a very narrow range of values for the usual socio-economic factors. Moreover, these demographic differentials are found to remain even when looking at socio-economic categories within each regional group. This point is discussed more fully later on; here I instead point to other studies (for example, Dyson and Moore 1983; Cleland 1985; Coale and Watkins 1986) which suggest strongly that cultural background has an important independent relationship to fertility and mortality in India as well as in other cross-cultural situations.

In seeking to understand what it is about a region or culture that might have this influence on birth and death rates in the Indian context, I draw on the Princeton European Fertility Project (see Coale and Watkins 1986). First, there is language: the North is predominantly Hindi-speaking, whereas the people of Tamil Nadu speak Tamil. But in the Indian case, it appears likely that language is merely a proxy for other aspects of the social structure and cultural identity rather than being in itself a determinant of demographic differentials through acting as a common medium for the spread of ideas. One can infer this from the fact that (especially in the urban environment discussed in this book), there are no Tamil-specific messages that users of that language alone can understand and accept. If anything, information tends to spread through the national language (especially in Delhi), which is Hindi; and, in any case, most of our South Indian respondents are bilingual. Rather than language being important because of the ease of information flow, as some writers have suggested, I would agree with Anderson (1986) that it is the identification with a linguistic group rather than the knowledge of a language which is the crucial factor.

Then much has been said about the role of religion in determining the timing of the fertility transition in different parts of Europe (see, for example, Livi-Bacci 1971; Lesthaeghe 1977). In the present context, religion is again a less important factor because both our cultural groups are largely Hindu and because the Hindu religion has no special views on procreation and birth-control, beyond the religious obligation to produce sons, which is independent of the culture studied.

Finally, one can bring in the physical characteristics of a region. It is conceivable that the conditions of life in one area (as defined

by climate, soil quality, and such factors) require different reproductive strategies for survival and progress from those in another
area. But this kind of hypothesis seems untenable in any direct
sense (although one can see it operating historically to institution-
alize fertility norms) because we know of no such physical
differences today and because cultural differentials in demographic behaviour tend to persist even among groups removed
from their original environment, as in the urban study.

What then is it that is culture- or region-specific in the Indian
context that might have an effect on fertility and mortality and
on their proximate determinants? Once more, we look at the
historical European experience and cite Knodel and van de Walle
(1986), 'One cultural feature that we believe the historical record
suggests as particularly important is the status of women. We
regard this more as a cultural characteristic than a socio-economic
or structural one since the extent to which women participate
in the broader socio-economic system beyond the home and
extended family appears to be determined more by religious
and other cultural values than by socio-economic development
per se.'

The next section of this chapter expands on the original and
modified motivations for the present study. It charts the evolution
of a concern with the cultural determinants of child mortality to
a broader and more useful look at demographic behaviour in
general. The interrelationships between mortality and fertility
provide the rationale for the new approach. Sections 1.2 and
1.3 plunge into a description of field methods. These sections
seem justified not only because they provide the context in which
discussions in subsequent chapters may be placed, but also because they afford an insight into a particular kind of field research,
one which lies somewhere in between an impersonal large-scale
survey and an individual anthropological investigation. In particular, section 2.3 should be read as a first-hand account of the kind
of stumbling-blocks that such fieldwork faces in a typical poor
country setting and, more importantly, of the unique satisfactions
that it also affords.

Chapter 2 sketches the field area and the various groups of
members of the study population. This is done to aid a more
qualitative understanding of the demographic analyses in later
parts of the book. Indeed, such a qualitative method is evident

throughout the book and should be treated as a reflection of the insights that descriptive analysis can offer as well as of the difficulties in quantifying some of the important findings of the study. However, it should be stressed that the main effort is to tease out quantitative relationships, and outcome measures in particular are largely quantitative.

Chapter 3 dissects the concept of women's status to seek measures of it which are most relevant to demographic behaviour. It latches on to three such measures: the extent of women's exposure to the world outside the home; the extent of their active (especially economic) interaction with this extra-domestic world; and the extent of their autonomy in decision-making. These measures are relevant to a range of cultural and geographical contexts. They are in turn related to two specific aspects of the North and South Indian culture: marriage and kinship systems, and women's economic roles. Chapters 4, 5, and 6 then go on to try to understand why and how these measures of women's status should have an effect on, respectively, fertility, child mortality, and gender differences in physical welfare.

The quantitative analyses are simple and much stress is laid on interpretations based on qualitative observations. This is partly because the qualitative field data offer richer interpretative possibilities than sophisticated statistical analyses in the framework of the present study. In particular, our measures of the status of women are indicative of female status (and, especially, female seclusion) rather than being the main feature of such status or seclusion. Indeed, as Chapter 3 brings out, they often cannot be ranked on a linear scale. It is therefore difficult to seek a direct relationship between every indicator of female status and demographic behaviour.

The one indicator of women's status which does seem to have general value is employment. And we do find that it is important at both macro and micro levels of analysis. At a community or macro level, it is found that there are links between demographic behaviour and levels of female employment when one compares cultural groups which differ on the latter variable. At an individual level, if employment is treated as a measure of seclusion, it is possible to demonstrate a relationship with fertility and with the sex differential in welfare. However, the female employment–child mortality relationship results are clouded by the negative impact of women's work on child survival due to a physical incompatibility between work and child-care.

Chapter 7 ties the strings together. It ends with a discussion of some of the policy implications of the study findings and a re-view of the generalizability of these findings. The impatient reader is directed to this last chapter for a flavour of the book as a whole.

1.1. Evolving Motivations

This study began with what seemed on the surface to be a very simple focus: the attitudinal and behavioural correlates of child health and mortality, the mother being the individual whose attitudes and behaviour were hypothesized to be major influences on these variables. The motivation for the study was the many recent analyses seeking to demonstrate the role of parental (or, more specifically, maternal) behaviour in child mortality. At one extreme, some of these analyses present the view that high levels of child mortality may be consciously maintained by parents to mitigate the effects of high fertility (see, for example, Scrimshaw 1978) or the observation that in nineteenth-century England poorer parents had a direct financial interest in the deaths of their babies as, for sixpence a week, it was possible to insure a child at birth for £5 to be paid at death (Ware 1977).

More generous and more frequent demonstrations of maternal attributes as important factors in child mortality have focused on the relationship between specific maternal characteristics and childhood mortality levels. And the characteristic most consis-tently observed to show a significant effect on child mortality has turned out to be maternal education. This relationship seems to hold not just when the data from recent surveys such as the World Fertility Survey are examined (for example, Caldwell 1981; Arriaga 1980), but even in more localized studies conducted several years ago (for India, see, for example, United Nations 1961; Driver 1963) as well as in studies of historical trends (for example, Basu 1987).

Having established that such maternal characteristics are corre-lated with child mortality, the next step is the attempt to identify the intermediate mechanisms through which this relationship operates. Especially important is the need to check whether maternal attributes are merely a proxy for household or even community or regional socio-economic circumstances in general, or whether such attributes also directly influence the proximate determinants of child mortality independently of household or environmental status. That this second pathway does function in an important way is suggested strongly by another source of evidence: data on sex differentials in child mortality in several South Asian countries. These data imply that, contrary to the experience in other parts of the world, in these countries girls have higher rates of mortality than boys and that this situation is changing only slightly in spite of steadily declining overall child-hood mortality levels. This kind of sex differential in mortality is 'artificially' maintained if one accepts the proposition that male children are biologically less hardy than female children. More-over, they point to the involvement of behavioural factors at the family level, as more impersonal influences from the outside should affect males and females in the same way, or even affect male children more adversely if they are inherently less resistant.[3]

The evidence implicating the household and especially the mother in child mortality is further strengthened by the observation that in India there are significant regional and cultural variations not just in overall levels of childhood mortality, but also in the extent of the sex differential in child death-rates. These regional variations are best expressed by dividing the country into northern and southern regions as has been done by several writers (e.g. Miller 1981; Dyson and Moore 1983). The states in the North are characterized not just by higher levels of childhood mortality but also by greater differences in male–female child death-rates as seen in the last two columns of Table 1.1.[4]

But much of the material on the subject of behavioural mechan-isms involved in child and especially female mortality tends to be limited in scope when in the urban areas,[5] or qualitative to the point of being anecdotal when in rural areas. While it is certainly very interesting and provides several pointers to further research, this kind of material cannot provide a basis for more rigorous cross-cultural comparisons because of this descriptive focus and/or because the independent studies of different cultural groups tend to have too many differences in their definitions and

Introduction

Table 1.1. Regional differentials in fertility,
childhood mortality, and the sex ratio of childhood mortality

State	Total fertility rate[a]	q(5)[b]	Sex ratio (male/female) of $q(5)$
North			
Haryana	4.5	.138	0.82
Madhya Pradesh	4.5	.197	0.96
Punjab	3.2	.111	0.88
Rajasthan	5.5	.176	0.89
Uttar Pradesh	4.3	.190	0.84
South			
Andhra Pradesh	3.2	.139	1.06
Karnataka	2.8	.142	1.02
Kerala	2.4	.080	1.12
Tamil Nadu	3.0	.132	1.02

[a] The Total fertility rate represents the total number of children that would have been born alive per woman had the current schedule of age-specific fertility rates been applicable for the entire reproductive period.

[b] q(5) represents the life-table probability of children dying between birth and exact age five.

Sources:

(1) Registrar General of India (1988), *Census of India 1981: Fertility in India,* Government of India, New Delhi.

(2) Registrar General of India (1988), *Census of India 1981: Child Mortality Estimates of India,* Government of India, New Delhi.

frameworks of analysis. Furthermore there are no controls for non-behavioural variables such as the external environment. There is also the disadvantage that most of the existing studies have tended to concentrate on the attitudes and practices of the upper caste (and class) groups, which are not numerically large enough to account by themselves for the regional variations in child and female mortality.

The present study intended to make a more quantitative assessment of the mechanisms through which differences in child mortality levels and in the sex ratio of child mortality are obtained in two culturally distinct sample populations, one North Indian and the other South Indian, but both now living in the same locality (to minimize the influence of non-behavioural factors). It was felt that such an analysis of the culturally influenced attitudinal and behavioural correlates of childhood mortality would also go a little way towards elucidating the mechanisms involved in the links between childhood mortality and maternal characteristics in general, because it was hypothesized that the position of women was one of the central variables in the relationship between cultural or regional background and the proximate determinants of infant and child mortality.

However, it soon became clear that one could not very well analyse child deaths without considering child births as well. The same forces which led to cultural variations in the one appeared to cause cultural differences in the other too. And all three (that is, these nebulous cultural forces, child mortality, and fertility) seemed to be linked in a tangle which would be the despair of any purist. Almost in mid-stream, we therefore cast the net a little wider. It now became important to examine the relationships between culture on the one hand and the range of demographic behaviour on the other. But it was decided that, although the data were available from the study, topics such as migration and to some extent marriage would be considered more marginally for the present. One did not want to be in the laughable situation of Professor Philip Swallow (mercifully only in a novel; see Lodge 1984), who, when asked to prepare a talk on literature and history, or literature and society, or literature and philosophy, or literature and psychology, for a British Council sponsored tour of Turkey somehow missed the 'or's in his telegram of invitation and made an idiot of himself (quite apart from the hours of backbreaking work which ruined all the fun of the trip) by taking on the relationship of not one but each and every one of these vast disciplines with literature.

To return to the revised objectives of the present study, the focus was now on culture and three aspects of demographic behaviour: childhood mortality, the sex differential in child health and mortality, and fertility. An attempt would be made to identify and describe some of the proximate determinants which were important in explaining cultural variations in these three variables, cultural variations being defined as those existing between a sample from North India and one from South India, two areas which have been found to differ greatly in broadly defined cultural characteristics (for a discussion of various such characteristics, see, among others, Karve 1965; Sopher 1980; Dyson and Moore 1983).

But culture is a catch-all term and obviously needs some definitional refinements if the relations between culture and demographic behaviour are to be of academic as well as policy interest. For it is not a particular language or religion or geographic area that in itself tends towards high or low fertility or mortality. These indicators of cultural identity serve as proxies for more specific characteristics of the people involved in these fertility or mortality levels. Here we took a lesson from the recent analytical interest in maternal attributes (especially education) and fertility and child mortality, as well as recent findings from historical demography, and decided to investigate empirically:

a. if cultural background is an important determinant of demographic behaviour;
b. if so, whether the position of women is an important component of cultural background which is responsible for this effect;
c. what the intermediate variables or proximate determinants of the link between women and demographic behaviour might be.

'Culture' was defined as a set of beliefs and practices common to a group defined by characteristics, such as region or language, other than the standard economic and social variables. That is, cultural practices and beliefs are those that transcend socio-economic differentials to embrace a whole regional group for example, and, conversely, tend to differ between different regional groups of similar socio-economic status.

So, finally, the more specific focus of this study became the relation between the status of women and demographic behaviour and that between cultural or regional background and the status of women. Of course there are several other important influences on fertility and (especially) mortality, not least the extra-household environment, both physically and in terms of the facilities and services available. For various reasons, this environment is also region-specific on many counts, hence one needed to control it if one wished to look at the women's status aspect of culture and its impact on demographic behaviour. Household socio-economic circumstances too may show regional propensities (for example, through regional differentials in income or occupational patterns) and we decided to control for this as well by limiting our study to the lowest rungs of the socio-economic ladder.

To ensure all the above controls, the study was therefore conducted among two sample populations, one of North Indian and the other of South Indian origin, but both now residing in the same environment, in this case a large resettlement colony or slightly upgraded slum in the city of Delhi. Co-residence in this slum took care of possible contamination of our results by both environmental as well as socio-economic differentials in our two cultural groups; all our households shared the same (generally insanitary) environment and the same constant need for a little more money just to keep going.

1.2. The Field Method

As already stated in the introduction, the present survey was concerned with examining in the field some of the cultural influences on demographic behaviour. Migrant households from the southern state of Tamil Nadu and the northern state of Uttar Pradesh were chosen to represent the northern and southern regions of India which have been described as being culturally distinct by several observers.

The actual field survey consisted of four parts:

1. Household listing: This constituted the first phase of the study and involved the listing of every household in the study area. The main reason for this was to identify the households from the regions we were interested in—the districts of Pratapgarh and Jaunpur in eastern Uttar Pradesh and the districts of Salem, South Arcot, North Arcot, and Madurai in Tamil Nadu. This listing process was also very useful in familiarizing the field-workers with the study area and making their presence more acceptable and welcome.

2. Canvassing of the household schedule: The household questionnaire was designed to collect basic socio-economic and demographic information from the sample households. It was administered to the heads of household by male interviewers and collected data on income, assets, migration details, recent births and deaths, and several general health-related household prac-

tices. In addition a complete listing of members was prepared for each household, with details of their birth, migration, educational, occupational, and marital circumstances. At this stage, the survey covered 976 households from Uttar Pradesh and 614 from Tamil Nadu.

3. Canvassing of the women's schedule: The women's questionnaire was administered by female interviewers to all ever-married women below the age of 60 in the sample households. It covered 642 women from Uttar Pradesh and 578 from Tamil Nadu. It was modelled broadly along the lines of the World Fertility Survey Core Questionnaire but also included important sections on female autonomy, knowledge, attitudes and behaviour on matters related to health and family planning, and attitudes and behaviour on matters related to the position of women. A detailed maternity history was obtained and for living children below the age of 12, information on their daily routine (for example, school attendance and work participation) was also obtained. Finally, during this retrospective survey, the heights and weights of the female respondents as well as of their children below 12 years were also recorded.

4. Longitudinal morbidity survey: This phase lasted for six months. All households with two or more living children below the age of 12 were visited once in two weeks to obtain ongoing information on the health status of these children. Incidents of illness were recorded using the WHO (1978) guidelines for the lay reporting of health information and elaborate details were gathered about the handling of such episodes of illness—the kind of medical care sought, the duration of illness, the diet during illness and convalescence, the child-care provider during the illness, and the number of missed days of school, work, or other normal activities. In addition, for each child in this sample, food consumption and school attendance details were obtained, the former by the method of previous day's recall and the latter with reference to the last two weeks. These last data provided very interesting information on regional differences in dietary practices which have a bearing on health in general and on sex differentials in health and well-being in particular. Since the data in the longitudinal study were obtained mainly from mothers, the female interviewers who did the retrospective female interviews were the investigators here as well. The longitudinal survey

covered 1055 children from Uttar Pradesh and 523 from Tamil Nadu.

All three questionnaires were extensively pre-tested before finalization. Especially important was the need to make the questions retain the exact sense, not just the flavour, of the original once they had been translated into Hindi and Tamil, the native languages of our two groups of respondents. Even after such pre-testing, several questions especially in the female schedule, were deliberately left uncoded and the interviewers were told to record the exact verbal replies received. Such responses were finally coded only after all the possible responses had been ascertained and some general judgements made. In fact, for each schedule the formal question-and-answer sessions were supplemented by much personal observation in the field by the interviewers as well as the study organizers. Indeed, the ability of the principal investigators to participate fully in the survey and collect much anthropological-type information was one of the more practical reasons for the choice of Delhi as the locale for the study. The interviewers were also encouraged to make copious notes on each interview and record verbatim any interesting responses that they received.

The field staff selected for the study were, as already mentioned, male for the household questionnaire and females for the female and morbidity questionnaires. Educationally, they all had at least a graduate degree in the social sciences, and in fact several of them had a post-graduate qualification as well. In addition the interviewers themselves belonged to the same two regions of origin as the respondents. This meant that they were able to talk to the households in their mother tongue and were also able to establish a better rapport with these households. The interviewers received intensive training in field procedures and in the details of the questionnaires they used. They were also actively involved in the process of translating the questions into Hindi and Tamil. Their work was supervised thoroughly in the field by a team of two field supervisors who allotted their work for the day and also monitored their performance through random re-interviews they conducted themselves.[6]

However, all this effort in planning and implementation was, we believe, well worth it because the data collected appear to be of overall good quality. There were problems in the field of course, and in the next section some of the more general of these problems are discussed both because they throw better qualitative light on the cultural context of the study and because at least some of the issues raised are relevant to other similar kinds of field-based research.

1.3. Some Field Problems and their Solution

In a very interesting evaluation of the Gambian census, Gibril (1979) states that in the course of obtaining and recording information, errors may result from the interviewer's inability to transmit what is wanted to the respondent, from the respondent not understanding the question, from the respondent's inability to provide the required information, from his method of conveying this information to the interviewer, and from the interviewer misunderstanding or misrecording the information given.

While it is true that in a sufficiently large census or survey such errors tend to cancel each other out, it is probably also the case that the nature and extent of an error is specific to a cultural or socio-economic context, so that analytical results of disaggregated groups give biased results. This is an important consideration in, for example, the cross-cultural analyses conducted by the World Fertility Survey, where identically framed questionnaires could still be getting somewhat different responses in different groups even when the actual correct answer expected is exactly the same. It is unfortunate that while so much effort has gone into method-ologies for analysing defective data there has been less practical concern with the possible defects themselves and how best they can be avoided at the stage of data collection. The only exception is age, where the difficulty of obtaining correct values in most traditional cultures has been repeatedly emphasized in the litera-ture. However, this emphasis did not stop the World Fertility Survey from insisting on all live births being given a year and month of delivery (and perhaps it was right; Preston (1985) for example, feels that the WFS procedure of imputing random dates of birth has not seriously affected the quality of data on birth intervals and child mortality).

The following paragraphs briefly discuss the main ways in which data collection posed problems in the present survey and some of the important means by which these were handled. We mention both general problems of field procedure and problems encountered in collecting specific kinds of information. In the latter case, in addition to those respondent-derived errors mentioned by Gibril, we consider the errors resulting from an unwillingness of the respondent (as distinct from his or her inability) to provide the correct information. Such unwillingness was an important variable during the pre-testing and early parts of the survey and although we usually managed to overcome it, in the case of a few kinds of information some questions had to be abandoned altogether.[7] The bulk of our observations relate to the pre-test and practice stages of the survey, since the manageable sample size, the small physical area covered, and the continuous monitoring possible because the study was based in Delhi, which is where the field staff and principal investigators lived, allowed us to identify and overcome most of these possible data biases in the field itself.

Accessibility and Co-operation

Accessibility and co-operation refer to two distinct concepts here. The first term is concerned with the actual physical availability of the respondent while co-operation refers to the rapport between the interviewer and interviewee once such contact has been established.

Strangely, physical accessibility in our study area posed two extreme problems—either the respondents were too easily available or they were not available at all. The former problem occurred especially with the female respondents from Uttar Pradesh. We certainly saw them, but rarely alone. Once the men had departed for the day, the women, who seldom work outside the home, emerged from their tiny and cramped quarters to gather in small groups in the narrow lanes outside their doors to continue with a host of household chores from chopping vegetables to combing children's hair and to enjoy simultaneously the one activity which makes the dullest tasks easy to finish: gossip and general verbal interaction with other women of their own cultural background.

Such pleasant meetings were often difficult to break up and it took a lot of persuasion to get a woman to re-enter her home for an interview in private. But once this feat had been achieved, it was usually possible to talk to the woman in peace for the hour or more that was required to fill in each questionnaire. There were certainly younger offspring clinging to their mothers' skirts, but fortunately for the survey, high male employment rates and the predominance of the nuclear family meant that we were free of the two relations most likely to influence a woman's responses to our questions: the husband and the mother-in-law. We adopted one further strategy to ensure spontaneous replies. A group of inter- viewers would descend on each lane together, so that all the women in one friendly circle could be interviewed simultaneously (but separately), thereby preventing a comparison of notes and anticipated questions (and therefore pre-planned answers) among the women who were interviewed later. This strategy was possible mainly because the women mixed most freely only with their immediate neighbours who, because of a residential clustering of families from the same region, were most likely also to belong to the same socio-cultural background.

The women from Uttar Pradesh were also the most likely group to be unavailable for days at a time because they had returned to their place of origin for a visit. As discussed elsewhere (Basu, Basu, and Ray 1987) in our study, the Uttar Pradesh migrant house- holds' links with the native village were much stronger than those of our South Indian sample. These links were maintained by either leaving the wives and children behind in the village, or else sending them back whenever possible. This generally meant that several of the women were away from Delhi during their children's summer holidays, which also coincided with the harvesting season at home, so that the additional labour was doubly welcome. Such absences from Delhi did not affect the retrospective part of our survey but was admittedly responsible for several cases from the North Indian sample being coded 'non-response' during the six-month longitudinal morbidity study.

The women from Tamil Nadu and the men from both regions were also difficult to interview if they were regularly employed. Such employment meant that they had to be contacted in the early mornings before they left for work or in the late evenings after they returned. The men were also often interviewed at the weekend as they usually hold jobs in the organized sector and get at least their Sundays off. For the South Indian working women, however, there is no such respite, as the majority of them work as domestic servants in the centre of the city and leave home as early as 6 a.m.; nor do most have even one weekly holiday. But this group of respondents turned out to be the most co-operative category and willingly spoke to our interviewers in the evenings even when this meant an interruption of their household chores. In fact it was common for an interviewer to accompany such a woman to the ration shop or the vegetable market and talk as they walked.

Indeed, it should be recorded that such unorthodox methods of data collection earned the interviewers a lot of goodwill and went a long way towards allaying respondents' natural suspicions. In addition, the evening interviews gave us an excellent opportunity to study the dramatic change in the character of the slum at this time. The change was especially noticeable in the role of women. No longer were the groups of gossiping North Indian women to be seen sunning themselves in the lanes. They had all retreated indoors, their place being taken by groups of idle men smoking and discoursing on the world after a long day in some distant work-place. Such idleness was quite understandable when one considered the mode of travel to and from work, either hanging precariously out of an overcrowded public bus, or, more commonly, negotiating a bicycle through loud streets of overbearing traffic. In the South Indian community, however, the women were completely visible in the evenings, often oblivious of the lounging men. In fact some of the more enterprising ones exploited the presence of the men and even ventured into the North Indian areas to sell the ethnic home-made snacks which they had spent all afternoon preparing. The only feature of slum life which did not change with the hour of the day was the ubiquitous presence of children, who ran freely through the streets whatever the time.

Co-operation was not at all uniform to begin with, and establishing a slow rapport with the initially suspicious respondents turned out to be an essential and eventually very gratifying part of the fieldwork. The first process of listing all the households in the area (so that those coming from our study regions could be identified) worked to our advantage as it gave us an opportunity to explain our motives and prepare people psychologically for the detailed surveys which followed and continued for the next 8 months. This initial contact with the residents, together with a pre-testing of the questionnaires in a similar slum nearby, also allowed us to anticipate potential bottlenecks in our survey design, make friends with some of the community leaders in the area, and generally become familiar and trusted faces in the locality.

A small incident well illustrates the initial hostility that is common in a migrant group in a new environment. During the household listing, the interviewers had been asked to record the times at which the men (and working women) were most likely to be found at home, so that we could schedule our interviews accordingly. This led a group of young men to publish a letter to the editor of the city's main Hindi newspaper wanting to know what innocuous motive a survey could have which wanted to catch the women alone at home and therefore enquired (conversely to our actual field question) when the men would be away. The tone of the letter made it clear that the authors did not expect our staff to settle for anything less than a rape, burglary, or forced sterilization.

Other fears and suspicions were more legitimate. The slum had recently been the centre of the worst post-assassination communal riots that followed the death of the then Prime Minister Mrs Indira Gandhi. For some days after the killing there had been virtual anarchy in the area, with several lives lost as well as much arson and looting. Since we entered the field only a few months after this event, there was some apprehension that we had come to enquire into the circumstances of the riots, identify the guilty, and probably even indict the innocent. Such fears led to an initial reluctance especially to answer questions on assets and belongings in case an attempt was made to imply that any particular possession had been acquired through stealing during the riots.

Then, there was the fear that our detailed fertility histories were in the nature of a stocktaking before restarting the compulsory sterilizations which several of these slum-dwellers vividly remembered from the Emergency days,[8] either through actual experience or through hearsay or, at times, through dramatically exaggerated rumours. Finally, there were the petty criminals—those with an illegal electricity connection, or an extra and false name in the family's ration card—who were wary of any detailed questions on their socio-economic situation.

However, these were all teething troubles and soon overcome.

Basically, they were overcome by the essentially trusting nature of the respondents, who were quick to believe and accept our stated motivations for doing the survey. Surprisingly, an academic motivation not connected with any action (especially governmental) agency was found to be an honourable and laudable aim by most families, especially by the women, indicating once more that anything to do with education quickly seems to acquire a high value in any group even superficially exposed to the outside world. Of course a few of the sharper residents wondered of what use such academic exercises finally were to the real world and its problems, but fortunately even such sceptics did not let their scepticism stop them from being ideal survey respondents.

Besides a generally friendly study population, a judicious mix of the following strategies seems to have accounted for the very satisfactory nature of the field-work:

1. Careful selection of the right kind of field interviewer: Besides the minimum educational qualifications (in this case, a degree in the social sciences), we found that the personality of the field-worker was an important determinant of performance. All our successful interviewers seemed to have an innate ability to communicate freely with people from any socio-economic class. Of course, it also helped that they spoke the same regional language as the respondent households. In addition, in the case of female interviewers, the ones who were accepted best were those who were married themselves or at least old enough to talk about fertility and family-planning matters with confidence. Initially we experimented woefully with a single girl just out of her teens who was shooed out of homes the minute she began to mention any method of contraception in an unsure, trembling voice. All our interviewers were also able to handle with great confidence the initial 'eve-teasing' (this peculiar Delhi term refers to the verbal and sometimes physical harassment of women by men) to which they were subjected when they passed through a lane, especially in the evenings. Such teasing stopped soon enough though, and in no time at all the young women had become respected and accepted daily visitors to the slum. Finally, our experience suggests that for the South Indian sample at least, the rapport between interviewer and respondent was greater because the majority of the Tamil interviewers belonged to the Brahmin or uppermost caste while the majority of Tamil

respondents belonged to the lower castes. We have discussed the homophilic versus heterophilic change agent in the context of family planning elsewhere (Basu and Sundar 1988) and will only note here that our respondents seemed to equate caste superiority with superiority in all matters and went out of their way to be co-operative and frank with the Brahmin interviewers.

On the whole, the female interviewers were able to establish much stronger roots in the local community than the male investigators, who had a relatively high turnover rate and were also less personally involved with the households they encountered. However, they were essential for the interviews with male heads of household, who would have looked askance at a young woman questioning them about their social and economic conditions.

2. Recruitment of local community leaders: Every such migrant slum throws up a few enterprising individuals who have the confidence and ability to act as middlemen between the slum-dweller and the outside world. Such interactions with the outside world are needed for a variety of aspects of day-to-day life—for example, in getting a ration card, school admission, an electricity connection, even a job—and persons who are perceived as being successful in mediating such interactions soon become much sought after and respected members of the community. We took the help of three such leaders to legitimize our study and also help us in actually conducting it. One of these was a barber (who was so confident about his influential contacts that he was soon offering to get our investigators jobs which would pay them twice as much as a miserly research project). One was an ex-soldier and ex-schoolteacher who had given up a regular life-style for the pleasures of the bottle—an indulgence that was willingly paid for by the other inhabitants who exploited his confident use of the English language. (Incidentally, he and a few other such enterprising residents listed their occupation as 'social worker'.) The third was a woman who ran a government nursery-school in her home. All three individuals were extremely useful as a base for our survey. In addition to persuading reluctant households to participate in the survey, they assisted in locating and identifying sample households, their homes functioned as a store-room for our morbidity registers, weighing machines, and stationery, and provided a much-needed place for rest for our interviewers, especially during the hot summer months.

3. The taking of anthropometric measurements: One part of the study was concerned with taking height and weight measurements of women and of children below the age of 12 in the sample households. The general enthusiasm for these measurements took the field staff as well as the study organizers completely by surprise. Compared to the persuasion and explanation required to get the women and men (especially from the northern region) to participate in the survey and answer questions, the alacrity with which young and old (including several whose measurements were not part of our study at all) jumped on to our weighing scales was quite astonishing. In fact, we soon discovered that the taking of these physical measurements before canvassing the questionnaire earned us more goodwill and co-operation than all our hoarse declarations about the purely academic nature of our study and the absence of sinister intent to collect information on tax evasion and/or unbridled fertility.

4. Willingness to go beyond the questionnaire: In a sense this was not very difficult since qualitative observations formed an important part of the study. However, the interviewers, by training and by inclination, often went well beyond the minimum required by participating actively in the life of the study household, listening patiently to detailed life histories, gratefully accepting the tea, snacks, and (the ultimate and barely affordable status symbol) soft drinks that were offered, and providing several kinds of physical, but never financial, assistance and advice. In fact, direct financial help was never sought, and in the rare instances that it was offered the respondent families politely rejected it, however useful it might have been to them. Besides avoiding monetary inducements the interviewers had also been carefully trained to make no false claims and promises about the direct effects of the survey to the study area. This kind of honesty, besides eventually raising the interviewer's esteem in the area, also minimized the respondent's urge to give the kind of answers which would be most likely to lead to, say, a new school or hospital or personal loan.

All the above strategies went a long way towards refining the general quality of the data collected, but there were still some problems with specific kinds of data which are worth mentioning here. While these problems were mainly of data availability, there were also a few important conceptual problems involved which are probably relevant to field procedures in other developing countries as well.

Age

The difficulty of obtaining exact months and years of birth have been noted extensively in the literature and will only be discussed here in the specific context of our survey. On the whole it appeared that women could less confidently state their current age than their age at an important event such as marriage (which was often implicitly calculated from the positive or negative gap between marriage and menarche). We used these stated ages at marriage together with the gap between marriage and the birth of the oldest living child and the current age of this child, to determine an estimated age of each women and compared this with her reported age. Such a comparison found that the divergence between the reported age and the estimated age was greater among the older women—for 70 per cent of the women whom we estimated to be below the age of 20, there was no gap at all. Older women often responded to the question on age by asking the interviewer, 'How old do I look?'

Still, our data do suggest that in the urban context at least, age is not as meaningless a concept as it is often thought to be. Fully 44 per cent of our respondents stated what appeared to be a correct current age (that is, it coincided with our estimated age—unless of course it happened that the reported age was being calculated by the women by using the same components as those used by us to calculate an estimated age), and in a further 47 per cent of cases the gap between estimated and reported age was within five years.

Fertility and Mortality

Besides the problem of errors in data about births discussed, for example, in Brass (1978), there seems to us to be one more important way in which fertility and by extension child mortality estimates derived from surveys (or censuses) may be biased. This is the bias caused by the very concept of fertility itself. By convention, the fertility of a woman is measured by the number of live births she has had. A live birth may be possible to define quite precisely medically, but may be confused in many cultures, especially those with a heavy dependence on lay assistance during deliveries and/or high levels of perinatal mortality. While few women in any culture would characterize a pregnancy outcome within the first six months of a pregnancy as a live birth, from the seventh month upwards, if the result of a delivery is a dead child, it is often far from clear whether this should be classed as a live birth or a stillbirth. The distinction routinely taught to field interviewers that a live birth is one in which the baby shows any signs of life after delivery, when explained to a respondent while discussing an event which she would best like to forget, is apt to be interpreted by her to rationalize her already firm beliefs about the matter. From our experience during the pre-test, a woman who is convinced (or has convinced herself) that her child died at birth because of medical or other third-party negligence is going to stick to her description of that event being a live birth, even in the face of a doctor's certificate stating that she had a stillbirth. On the other hand a grieving woman with real or imagined feelings of guilt about a child that died very soon after birth is equally likely to insist that the baby was dead in the womb, a view that will often be sympathetically supported by the midwife and other relatives present during the delivery. Finally, besides these two kinds of women who choose not to probe too deeply into the truth about a pregnancy outcome, there is also the third kind who genuinely does not know whether she had a stillbirth or a live birth.

While it is true that the above biases in reporting of stillbirth can work in opposite directions and may even cancel each other in a large sample so that final fertility estimates remain reasonably accurate, it is possible for the bias to operate in a single direction for different sub-groups of a population. For example, Ware (1984) describes how many African groups define any child that dies before passing through the 'outdooring' ceremony (which takes place about a week after birth) as a stillbirth. From all this, one wonders if it might not have been better if convention had defined fertility in terms of number of pregnancies which progress to the seventh month rather than those which result in a live birth.

Then, there is the culture-specific tendency to omit dead children in maternity histories. While a certain amount of this is probably really a question of faulty recall, it may also sometimes be a genuine reluctance to discuss an unfortunate event. Moreover, dead children at the early reproductive stage are particularly difficult to recall by women with several subsequent births, so that women with high fertility will be precisely those whose fertility is underestimated. But whatever the cause, the effect on analytical findings is worse when the omission of child deaths is selective in some way. For example, in our sample, in spite of our best efforts, the birth histories of women gave us a sex ratio of live births of 114 for the Uttar Pradesh respondents and 103 for the Tamil Nadu mothers. There was thus obviously a significant under-reporting of dead daughters by the North Indian women and this should clearly be noted when discussing the strong female disadvantage in survival which was apparent for the Uttar Pradesh households even from the reported births.

Knowledge, Attitudes, and Practice of Family Planning

Not surprisingly, this is the section in demographic surveys which has received the greatest amount of flak. We mention here only a few specific problems with data collection on this topic, which appear to be common to all South Asian cultures.

First, there is the unfair insistence in most surveys on a numeric response to all questions where a numerical answer is conceivable. Take ideal family size, for example. The problems inherent in this concept have been succinctly discussed in Lightbourne and MacDonald (1982), who then go on to say that the WFS experience suggests that, with sufficient probing, it is possible to obtain numerical answers from respondents who initially give a non-numeric response. This is why the WFS 'Interviewers Instructions' directed interviewers to press for a numeric response to questions on total number of children desired and additional number of children wanted. But is this wise? In Bangladesh, for example, in spite of such insistence by the interviewer, as many as 29 per cent of respondents gave non-numeric responses to the question on total number of children desired, forcing Thompson, Ali, and Casterline (1982) to conclude that such non-numerical answers are as legitimate and meaningful as clear numeric replies. And in the other countries where Lightbourne and MacDonald did find low levels of non-numeric answers, one wonders how many of the resulting answers are statements of real views and how many are due to a resignation to interviewer pressure. In our survey, there were interesting regional differences in the non-numeric responses on ideal family size. While about 10 per cent of the Tamil women gave such a response, for the respondents from Uttar Pradesh this figure was as high as 26 per cent. Obviously, treating this as a non-response is going to positively bias estimates of measures such as the unmet need for contraception, but differentially for the two regions so that comparisons become almost meaningless. In fact, what is more meaningful here is the regional differential in this so called non-response, rather than the differences in the numerical replies.

Questions related to family planning methods in general and those which involve any discussion of sexual behaviour in particular are also found to be, at least initially, difficult to ask in most South Asian cultures. In our study, we faced four distinct problems in this area:

(*a*) Due to the politicized sterilization programme of the mid-1970s, which several of our North Indian households remembered as discussed earlier, until our credentials in the field were well established, women were reluctant to talk about actual contraceptive use. However, this reluctance was soon overcome and does not in any way bias our results.

(*b*) In the section on contraceptive knowledge, several women mentioned 'injection' as a method of contraception. This has also been noted by the WFS in Bangladesh by Thompson, Ali, and Casterline (1982). However, we were not able to establish whether this mention was a reflection of a genuine knowledge of the method (caused for example by knowledge of a Depo-provera programme in a city government hospital) or of a hazy belief that there must be something like an injection to prevent births in the same way as preventing illnesses.

(*c*) There seemed to be a certain amount of embarrassment, especially among the women from Uttar Pradesh, in talking about views on and practice of post-partum and (especially) terminal abstinence, and we finally left it to the interviewer's discretion to ask questions on this matter only at the end of the interview and even leave out the questions altogether in cases where she felt that an insistence on replies would jeopardize the goodwill established during the rest of the interview. However, on reflection it now appears that this was an unduly stringent precaution on our part—

skilled interviewers were able to overcome any shyness on these issues relatively easily (as long as husbands or female relatives, not friends, were completely out of earshot), whereas some interviewers tended too readily to exercise the option not to ask these questions at all.

(*d*) Some of the respondents in their turn asked the field staff a lot of questions about family planning and some of the answers coded in the questionnaires could have been biased by the timing and nature of the information imparted by the interviewers—which could not always be rigidly controlled.

Socio-Economic Characteristics

The initial difficulties in obtaining information on income and assets have already been discussed in the earlier section on 'Accessibility and Co-operation'. In addition, we faced some other data-collection problems which were specific to the cultures we were studying but need to be mentioned here to illustrate the need to combine an intimate descriptive knowledge of a culture with quantitative survey methods, especially those with pre-coded questionnaires. For example, one unanticipated hurdle was the refusal of women in much of South Asia, and especially in northern India, to utter the names of their husbands. This common practice meant that the response to a request for a straightforward biographical detail such as 'wife of —', evoked either a stern silence from the older women or a shy giggle from the younger ones. This hurdle was fortunately easily removed by approaching either a neighbour or an older relative for a name or else by calling out the names of adult males listed in the household questionnaire and noting the one which elicited a nod of assent.

Then there was caste. Several social scientists have noted the tendency in India for the lower castes not only to ape the customs of the higher caste groups with social and economic mobility but also to seek a gradual affiliation with an upper caste. In our sample this tendency was greater in the South Indian households, but since the interviewers were also of the same cultural background they were easily able to distinguish, for example, between the few genuine Brahmin households and those that called themselves Brahmins because of greater economic prosperity.

Next, while the enthusiasm for anthropometric measurements was generally high as already discussed, there were also a few prejudices against such measurements in selected groups. For example, in the North Indian samples it was considered inauspicious for a pregnant woman to be weighed, while among the South Indians a child with an illness (especially chickenpox) was not allowed to be measured for fear of ill luck.

Finally, it is worth stressing once again that even a straightforward question and what seems an unambiguous answer might require non-standard interpretations in different socio-cultural contexts, which is why the present study laid so much emphasis on qualitative data collection as well. For example, we had several households whose members clearly stated that they had no electricity in the home, but who, in the section on assets, nevertheless claimed a television set (there are no battery-operated sets in India). The discrepancy was soon resolved when we realized that what these households meant was that they had no legal electricity connection; instead they (costlessly) made do with a long wire which tapped electricity from a nearby streetlight.

Similarly, in the maternity histories of women, we discovered that we had no code under 'current status of live birth' for a 'Don't know' response. In a small but noticeable number of cases the women genuinely did not know the whereabouts or survival status of a child which had simply disappeared. And for children of school age, under 'reasons for not going to school', our pre-test had missed out an important reason unconnected with parental wishes and resulting from the childhood anarchy common in urban slum life: 'the child refuses to go'. Then, in several cases the stated existence of the apparently harmful custom of delaying the onset of breast-feeding until the third or fourth day after birth actually meant that the biological mother did not breast-feed the baby but a surrogate did. In all such ambiguous cases, the field interviewers had been explicitly instructed to write down their findings in words and not mindlessly tick the closest coded answer and so we were fortunately able to take such unforeseen situations into account at the stage of data analysis.

NOTES

1. The Princeton European Fertility Project and the World Fertility Survey respectively.
2. Of course this is not to imply that the northern and southern parts of the country are themselves homogeneous. There are substantial differences, but for the purposes of our hypothesis, these are not significant.
3. There is also the finding that in most of the South Asian data, it is only after the first month or so (when maternal behaviour usually begins to exert a role) that female mortality overtakes male (see e.g. Arora, Prakasan and Karkal, 1979; Chen, Rahman, and Sardar, 1980). Neonatal mortality is generally greater for males than for females. This is in keeping with the fact that early infant mortality is more influenced by biological factors (and therefore favours girls) or due to non-discriminatory practices which result in a high proportion of neonatal deaths being caused by tetanus for example.
4. This geographical delineation is even more striking given the range of socio-economic conditions present in each region.
5. For example, studies showing more boys than girls among hospital admissions can be linked to unrelated field studies which find a higher incidence of illness or malnutrition among girls.
6. In addition, the field staff spent every Friday afternoon at the National Council of Applied Economic Research Head Office, where they discussed any problems they had faced, clarified doubts raised by the office staff during the editing of the previous week's output, and received any additional instructions.
7. See Bleek (1987) for a refreshingly honest appraisal of the high probability that a researcher will utterly fail to collect reliable information on a number of delicate matters which demographers routinely use as their variables. Some of the results of such statistical analyses based on direct data on culturally sensitive subjects rightly need to be taken with a pinch of salt.
8. This refers to the state of national emergency declared in India by the Indira Gandhi government during 1975–7. One of the disciplines sought to be imposed during this time was contraceptive acceptance, and in some parts of the country, mainly in North India, there was a short-lived attempt to increase sterilization acceptance through measures which crossed the thin line between persuasion and coercion.

2

The Field Area and
its Inhabitants

THIS chapter describes the physical and social environment of
the study area and provides short impressions of the sample
households in general and their female and child inhabitants in
particular. The former is important because it portrays the
background against which our demographic events occur and,
especially in the case of health and mortality, itself has an impact
on these demographic events. Moreover, it is shaped by the
specific cultural life-styles of its inhabitants and therefore comple-
ments the profiles which follow of the two regional groups in the
study.

2.1. The Study Area

The present survey was conducted in a large multicultural resettlement colony (which is for all practical purposes a slightly
glorified slum) situated in East Delhi on the newer and more
isolated side of the River Yamuna. The colony was set up during
the Emergency in the mid-seventies to house migrant squatters
from all over the city. There are three adjoining colonies on a total
area of abut 12.4 hectares.

All the households in this area belong to the lower social and
economic classes. They were provided with the minimum facilities
of public water and toilets and then left to do with their 25 square-
yard plots as they thought fit. Each household was also given a
small loan (of Rs 2000) to encourage them towards building a
habitable dwelling. The result is that about half the households
have built a permanent (in a few cases even two-storied) cement
structure, while the rest are content with a semi-permanent or
worse hut. Twenty-five square yards is not a large area and most
homes therefore consist of a solitary room for the conduct of all

household and even some business activities. However, as discussed later, much activity also spills out on to the narrow lanes between two rows of houses, so that in the daytime of the winter months at least, the seeker of privacy finds it relatively easy to be the sole occupant of his or her room for several hours at a stretch.

Housing Conditions

The colony we studied is divided into 36 blocks of about 500 plots each. The plots are arranged side by side with no open spaces in between in long rows of about 20 houses per row. With such overcrowding and the poorly ventilated structures that have been constructed (few homes boast more openings than a single door), it is not surprising that to most households these plots represent no more than a legal physical shelter. However, a few of the more enterprising residents have started small businesses in their rooms during working hours. These businesses include petty vending, tailoring, electrical repairs, and small-scale manufacture of various knick-knacks. One of the most common and popular of such enterprises is the setting-up by several of the women from Tamil Nadu of a kitchen in their homes to make popular regional snacks such as *dosas* and *vadas*, which they hawk in the by-lanes of the colony. Their buyers are far more eclectic than their cuisine, however, and in the early hours of the evenings, Rajasthanis and Punjabis can be seen devouring the delicacies with as much gusto as the Tamils.

It should also be mentioned here that though the colony is multicultural in the sense that it includes migrants from virtually every part of the country, the tendency is for households from the same region of origin to cluster together, so that we have whole lanes consisting of only Tamils or only Biharis, and so on. This seems to be the general pattern in slums all over the country (see de Souza 1978).

The colony is now much larger than originally planned, because of the influx of new arrivals from other parts of Delhi, as well as from other parts of the country. The households have migrated here for the public amenities that the place offers and because of kinship or other ties with the original households. The newcomers have set up their little huts in clusters around virtually every block and have been quick to seek to legitimize their position by employing every strategy to acquire that definitive proof of identity and residential status: the ration card.

Such uncontrolled expansion naturally means that the already meagre public facilities in the area are being severely strained, and such strain together with the daily life-style of the slum-dwellers has had its greatest negative impact on the general level of sanitation and hygiene in the area. This level is appallingly low and the dirt and squalor of the lanes and surroundings are in shocking contrast to the interiors of individual homes, which are often spotlessly clean in spite of the constraints on resources. A sparkling stainless steel utensil is the first symbol of such house pride and many homes estimate their welfare levels in terms of the number of such utensils that they can acquire. Such contradictions between household and social hygiene were well brought out in another Indian slum study (Shekhar 1983) in which homes were classified according to the levels of cleanliness of their interiors and immediate exteriors: 17 per cent of the homes were rated as poor on a scale of sanitary conditions inside them, while 40 per cent deserved a similar rating for conditions immediately outside the home.

The local government had made provisions in its planning of the area for schools, hospitals, markets, etc. and, as described below, several of these facilities have actually been realized. Yet this is not nearly enough. For example, every lane has one or two public water taps and every block has access to a row of public lavatories. In addition, some of the more affluent households have installed their own water supply in the form of a handpump outside their homes. However, there is no space for private bathrooms or toilets and even though there are public toilets near each block, not everyone (and certainly not young children) uses these. Even several of those who claim that they do use the public toilets actually mean that they squat outside the toilets rather than outside their homes. This is not so surprising when one considers that these toilets are often not cleaned regularly and do not have a sufficient water supply. Moreover, as discussed in later chapters, there are several cultural restrictions and security considerations which prevent women and (especially) adolescent girls from some regions from using the public toilets.

Another reason for the distressingly insanitary local environment is the garbage thrown all over the place. For this the blame lies partly with the municipality for not cleaning the streets or clearing the garbage dumps regularly and partly with the people who have little compunction about throwing rubbish outside their doors. In our sample households, for example, only about two-thirds of households from Uttar Pradesh reported that they threw their garbage in the official heap, while for the Tamil households this figure was somewhat higher at about 80 per cent.

Transport

The area is well connected to the city centre by the public transport system. Several buses start and terminate within the colony. But buses mean fares and many of our households have decided that it is more economical in the long run to invest in a bicycle to take the men to work. Several of the Tamil women who work as domestic servants in the city have also arranged a private chartered bus for themselves instead of trusting to the vagaries of the public bus, which is only marginally cheaper. The majority of children in the area do not require special transport arrangements as they either do not go to school at all or else go to the local government schools, which are all within easy walking distance. The only exceptions are those older Tamil children who go to the main Tamil-medium school in the centre of the city and for whom there is a regular school bus. The other popular mode of travel for short distances is the cycle-rickshaw. However, these are more useful to their owners than to commuters because they are used mainly by the affluent residents of newly constructed nearby neighbourhoods and therefore provide the household income to several residents of our study area.

Health

On paper at least, our study area appears to be well provided with medical services, one of the reasons being that the high density of these resettlement colonies has made their residents able to exert considerable political pressure, especially at election time. To begin with, the Municipal Corporation of Delhi runs a 28-bed maternity centre in another resettlement colony which is a couple of kilometres away from our slum. This centre handles simple deliveries, but complicated cases are referred to a general hospital some 10 km away.

In addition, in our study area itself, there are as many as five dispensaries (one of these is even a polyclinic—a clinic which is supposed to have specialists in several branches of medicine) run by various departments of the government, which are open to the general public. One of the medical colleges in the city as well as a social welfare organization have also set up permanent health camps in the area (mainly providing child health services). All these government or semi-government health centres are free in principle, but it must be added that they are chronically short of any but the most general medicines (such as pain-killers and skin ointments). Their working hours are also usually limited to the mornings and early afternoons, though one of the clinics becomes a homeopathic dispensary in the evenings. The local government also has an ayurvedic dispensary in the slum, thus paying more than lip-service to the policy of popularizing indigenous medicine (ayurveda is the ancient Indian system of medicine that relies primarily on the use of herbs and plants). In addition to the shortage of medicines and often inconvenient timings already mentioned, the other great drawback of these government clinics is that, although they are supposed to be staffed by a complement of three full-time doctors, rarely does a clinic have even two. Finally, seven dispensaries is not really all that large a figure given the size of the population they are supposed to serve—close to 175 000.

It is not surprising, therefore, that the area has seen a proliferation of private medical practitioners. There are about thirty licensed private practitioners in and around the colony and they typically charge a fee of Rs 5–10 for a consultation plus medicines (usually an injection). These doctors are generally open in the evenings and their main disadvantage is that they are predominantly male. It should also be added that it would perhaps be inaccurate to refer to these private practitioners as private physicians. The majority of those who have set up their clinics in our study area do not have a formal medical degree; instead they attach a string of cryptic qualifications such as GAMS and MIMS to their name-plates.

Finally, there are the traditional birth attendants or *dais*. Almost every block (that is, every cluster of 500 households) has one or two such midwives. These women usually belong to the lowest castes (mainly the sweeper caste) and come from the northern Indian states of Haryana and Uttar Pradesh. The occupation of midwife is hereditary, but business is now slacker than it used to be (many of them ruefully blame the maternity hospitals and the family planning programme for this), so they are often employed in other occupations as well, generally in domestic service. The typical *dai* does not provide any antenatal care; she is called in at the onset of labour, more or less takes charge of the actual delivery, and receives Rs 21 or 31 (even Rs 51 if the child is male) and gifts in kind for her services. Sometimes she provides post-natal care for about a month (primarily bathing the baby and massaging the new mother) in which case her fee can rise to Rs 101.

Besides these services in their immediate vicinity, all our respondent households also have access to the health facilities outside their residential area, of course. These services vary greatly in quality and quantity in different parts of the city, but the main conclusion is that, in principle, all our slum households have access to more or less equal services.

Education

As in the case of health, the educational facilities in our slum area are also impressive, especially on paper. To begin with, there are the *balwadis* or nursery schools run by the Delhi Council of Child Welfare. These charge a nominal fee of Rs 2 per month and besides some pre-school activities also provide lunch for the children. In spite of this, attendance remains very poor (rarely are more than 50 per cent of the children officially on the rolls present). In addition, the Integrated Child Development Scheme (ICDS) of the Government of India runs one *anganwadi* or pre-school centre per 1000 of slum population. This is staffed by local workers and provides supplementary nutrition, immunization, and health check-up services for children below the age of 6 as well as for nursing or pregnant women. In addition, children in the 3–6 years age-group receive some pre-school training. Once again, the services of these *anganwadis* tend to be grossly under-utilized even by working mothers.

The Municipal Corporation of the city also runs a number of primary schools in the area. These schools do not charge any fees and also supply the children with free books and one set of school uniform per year; this is obviously not enough, so the schools present a pleasantly colourful sight as the children generally attend in their non-school clothes. The schools also have a free midday meal scheme, but funds are insufficient for more than a couple of slices of bread for only a few months in the year. These schools officially have qualified trained teachers, but many parents complain about the poor quality of teaching and the need to spend money on private tuition either from these teachers themselves or from older students who take pupils to finance their own education. While most of these government schools have Hindi as the language of instruction, the Corporation has also started a Tamil-medium primary school in deference to the sizeable local Tamil population in the area.

The Municipal Corporation also runs two secondary and three senior secondary schools in the colony. These are all Hindi-medium schools and the products of the Tamil primary school have to seek (and often fail to obtain) admission in the major Tamil high school in the heart of the city, which has the funds to teach some of these poor students free of charge.

Entertainment

There is a cinema hall in the area showing regular Hindi films for nominal prices. Its popularity has waned somewhat with the rapid rise in the number of households who own television sets, so that many people can now watch either their own or a neighbour's. There are also several small temples in the colony and each regional group generally throws itself wholeheartedly into the celebration of all its ethnic festivals and ceremonies such as marriage. But our field experience suggests that by far the greatest amount of entertainment is provided by the neigh-bourhood gossip sessions which fill up all the leisure time of the men and even reduce the monotony of the daily household routine of the women. The small size and discomfort of homes is an advantage in this respect—very little excuse is needed to place a cot (a light bedstead) outside the door and gather in a small group to chat and while away the hours.

2.2. The Household Described
(Including a Note on the Migration Process)

As mentioned in the previous chapter, our sample households belonged to two regional groups, one North Indian and the other South Indian. The former consisted of 976 households from the south-eastern districts of Jaunpur and Pratapgarh in the state of Uttar Pradesh (eastern Uttar Pradesh is the more undeveloped and poorer part of the state) and the latter of 614 households from the districts of South Arcot, North Arcot, Salem, and Madurai in the state of Tamil Nadu. Except for the households from Madurai, which belong to a weavers' community, most of our respondents had been landless labourers or marginal farmers in their states of origin, driven to Delhi by variations on the theme of poverty. For some it was two years of successive drought, for others it was the loan taken after a bad harvest, still others would only say that they came to Delhi 'in search of employment'. As for the weavers from Madurai district, their break with a traditional profession and the move to Delhi were connected with the general, often precipitous, decline in the demand for their skills in the home village. In fact, many of the women from this community, who were skilled weavers at home and now work as domestic servants in the city, are still bitter about this shift to a menial occupation.

However, it should be noted that it is the men, especially the male heads of households, who stated such primarily economic motivations for migrating to Delhi. For women, the stated reasons for the move to Delhi were completely different. By far the most important cause of this move was either marriage or accompaniment of a migrating husband, with the next most popular answer being the accompaniment of migrating parents. Rarely did the South Indian women and never did the North Indian women decide independently to migrate to Delhi.

We now turn to the regional differential in the reasons for migration. As Singh (1984) points out, while it is true that most female migration in India is associated with or dependent on male migration, this is not a sufficient excuse to move in all cases. There is often a compelling secondary (economic) reason which clinches the issue. Women (and children) are more likely to move with the men if there is a greater possibility of their becoming economically productive after the move. This accounts at least partly for the inverse association between the sex ratio (males/females) of a migrant stream and female labour-force participation rates among migrants.

In our own study we found this secondary but nevertheless important economic motive for female migration reflected in three interrelated facts:

1. The migrants from Tamil Nadu were much more likely to have moved as family units rather than as (male) individuals than were those from Uttar Pradesh. In the former sample (which included all, not just a selection of, the households from the selected districts in Tamil Nadu in our study area) the sex ratio (males per 100 females) of the population was 103, while for the Uttar Pradesh sample it was much higher at 140. Indeed, 20 per cent of the households from Uttar Pradesh included no women, whereas the corresponding figure for the Tamil Nadu sample was 2 per cent. Moreover, in the latter case the men in the households without women were more likely to be unmarried or widowed, while a high 85 per cent of the men in the Uttar Pradesh sample households without women were currently married, that is, they had left their wives behind in the village. This kind of conjugal separation of migrants from northern India in general and Uttar Pradesh in particular has been noted by several researchers (see, for example, Mazumdar and Mazumdar 1976; Singh 1978; Banerjee 1984).

2. The women in the Tamil Nadu households in our study were much more likely to be employed then their North Indian counterparts. Only 46 per cent of the women aged 19–59 years in the former group were unemployed, this figure being close to 95 per cent in the northern Indian group.

3. Of the women aged forty and above, a much higher proportion (41 per cent) of the South Indian women were widows or divorced/separated than were the North Indians (14 per cent). This did not mean that the death or desertion rate of Tamil husbands was unduly high; it only meant that after such an event, the Uttar Pradesh women tended to leave the city and go back to the village of origin, whereas for the Tamil women such an event was not a call to pack up and go home, their relative economic and social independence making their move to the city as stable and permanent as that of the men with whom they originally came.

So the finding is that the North Indian women are not as economically motivated to migrate as the South Indian women, both because they do not consider the employment opportunities in the city attractive enough and (more importantly) because they belong to a culture of low female participation in the labour-force. On the other hand, our data support Singh and de Souza's (1980) finding that low caste and class Tamil migrant women frequently said that they believed that the woman had as much responsibility as the man to work and support the family.

One important consequence of this regional differential in the role of women and in the subsequent nature of the migration process has been that there are important regional differences in the extent of the break from the village of origin (see Basu, Basu, and Ray 1987). We found that a much larger proportion of the households from Uttar Pradesh than from Tamil Nadu maintained regular contact with the region of origin, sent money home, and themselves intended to return to their place of origin sometime in the future rather than settle down permanently in Delhi.

Life-styles and Socio-cultural Variation

Once our respondents have arrived in Delhi, we continue to find regional differences in several aspects of our groups' life-styles. The employment of women has already been mentioned. The other general difference was that, in spite of this higher level of female employment, on the whole the households from Tamil Nadu in our sample were worse off economically than those from Uttar Pradesh. Table 2.1 summarizes this regional differential in economic well-being. (This economic differential is also interesting because of the lower fertility and mortality in our South Indian sample which seem to exist in spite of their relatively greater poverty; see Chapters 4 to 6.) But whatever these differences, the similarities are greater. The biggest similarity is that all our respondent households belong to the lowest socio-economic classes. Yet we find interesting differences in several socio-cultural variables as seen in Table 2.2. To summarize, compared to Uttar Pradesh, the households from Tamil Nadu:

(*a*) exhibit lower fertility and therefore have fewer young children;

(*b*) in spite of (*a*) above, have a larger mean household size;

(*c*) are more likely to be of the extended or joint family type;

(*d*) are more likely to contain older members, that is, aged 60 years and above;

(*e*) have fewer remaining ties with the area of origin; and

(*f*) are more likely to do things as a united family group than as a

Table 2.1. Regional differentials in economic status

	Uttar Pradesh (N=976)	Tamil Nadu (N=614)
1. Mean monthly household income (Rs)	926	832
2. Mean monthly per capita income (Rs)	289	197
3. Mean number of rooms per household	1.54	1.37
4. Mean amount of money currently borrowed (Rs)	1153	1449
5. Per cent of homes with own water supply	35	22
6. Per cent of homes with an electricity connection	57	48
7. Per cent of homes with a solid cement structure	71	49
8. Per cent of household heads in regular salaried employment	86	61

group of hierarchical members (see row 6 of Table 2.2 for instance).

At first sight, the above might appear to be a ragbag of socio-cultural differences. But there is a clear chain linking these variables. Our overall picture is that because of the nature of the female role and the subsequent migration process, the households from Tamil Nadu are more likely to have migrated in family groups rather than as individuals, indeed the tendency is for these groups to contain members of extended, rather than nuclear, families. This means that there are already strong kinship ties in the city of arrival and therefore over time the village of origin holds fewer attractions. These family and kinship ties become, if anything, stronger in the new, often initially hostile, environ-ment, so that there is a tendency to function as a group in both living arrangements as well as in routine activities of day-to-day life. We would go a step further and add that this expression of greater intra-household unity and equality is also a result and not just a cause of the greater economic emancipation and autonomy

Table 2.2. Regional differentials in socio-cultural variables

	Uttar Pradesh (N=976)	Tamil Nadu (N=614)
1. Per cent of households which are nuclear	77	73
2. Mean household size	4.39	4.74
3. Mean number of children aged 0–14 years per household	1.94	1.87
4. Mean number of persons aged 60 and above per household	0.03	0.08
5. Mean number of earners per household	1.30	2.00
6. Per cent of housholds where all members eat together at the evening meal	50	76
7. Per cent of households that regularly remit money	30	6
8. Per cent of households that plan to return home one day	13	6
9. Per cent of households where any members smoke	79	68
10. Per cent of households where any members drink[a]	36	41

[a] We believe these figures to be gross underestimates.

in decision-making that the South Indian women enjoy. We discuss this question of the regional differential in the status of women repeatedly in the context of demographic behaviour in later chapters. Here we only mention that this impact of the position of women extends into several other areas besides those directly relevant to demographic behaviour, in particular into those areas directly concerned with the handling and facing of the situation of poverty.

2.3. The Woman Described

Since this entire monograph is built around the theme of cultural differentials in the position of women, a lengthy section 2.3 would involve repetition of material which is brought up in later chapters. So here we more or less content ourselves with Table 2.3, which provides a handy reference to the various indicators of our sample women's socio-economic and cultural circumstances that appear in different contexts on the following pages.

But a brief comment or two on some of the items in Table 2.3, especially those relevant to the issues of the status of women, cannot be resisted. First, there is the interesting regional differential in female employment (we ignore here the equally relevant differential in education because its implications for the position of women are more obvious). Not only are the women from Tamil Nadu much more likely to be working than those from Uttar Pradesh (with all the attendant implications for women's self-confidence and independence), the kinds of employment they tend towards are even more relevant to their position in general. On the whole, the women from Uttar Pradesh, if they earn an income at all are likely to do so by activities which involve the minimum interaction with the outside world and certainly virtually no interaction with men from the outside world. Almost all such employment is household-based and generally centres around traditional feminine skills such as sewing, food processing, or the manufacture of various knick-knacks for sale by others.

On the other hand, the women from Tamil Nadu are much more catholic in the kinds of employment they are willing to consider. They have fewer inhibitions about the interactions with the extra-domestic world that several types of work entail—indeed, our field observations suggest that they revel in such interactions, not least because of the much greater information for thought and for gossip that such interactions provide. As row 3 of Table 2.3 indicates, domestic service is the most popular form of employment for these women. Such employment, besides often being the first choice of the South Indian women for various reasons, also has a profound influence on their attitude to life (see Basu and Sundar 1988) and therefore deserves to be described in a little detail.

A typical domestic servant works seven days a week, six hours a day (to which must be added the, often considerable, travel time to and from work) and is employed in four or five homes to sweep and wash the floors, clean the dishes, and wash the clothes. For this, she takes home the equivalent of about £15 every month. In

Table 2.3. Regional differentials in the socio-cultural position of ever-married women

Socio-cultural variable	Uttar Pradesh (N=642)				Tamil Nadu (N=578)			
	Age-group of women				Age-group of women			
	15–29	30–49	50+	All ages	15–29	30–49	50+	All ages
1. Per cent women with some education	17	7	0	11	29	21	4	23
2. Per cent employed	3	8	13	6	58	75	52	65
3. Per cent working as domestic servants	0	0	0	0	52	58	38	53
4. Per cent educated women who are employed	4	29	0	11	45	73	50	56
5. Per cent uneducated women who are employed	2	7	13	5	64	75	52	67
6. Mean number of years of education of husbands	5.5	3.3	3.3	4.4	3.5	3.1	1.7	3.2
7. Per cent husbands with regular salaried jobs	78	92	74	85	69	52	34	59
8. Mean age at marriage	9.8	8.1	7.8	8.9	16.4	15.9	15.4	16.1
9. Mean age at cohabitation, following marriage	14.7	15.2	15.7	15.0	16.5	16.2	16.7	16.4
10. Mean gap in years between husband's and wife's age	4.8	4.1	3.6	4.4	6.3	7.5	8.3	7.0
11. Per cent households with a								
Television	17	14	19	16	14	19	10	16
Sewing-machine	23	21	33	22	7	11	4	8
Fan	2	3	0	3	2	3	2	2

addition, she also collects the occasional parcel of left-over food and receives clothes and other gifts during her employer's family celebrations. It must also be added that, in spite of the heavy inputs needed, the work is not all drudgery. There is usually enough time to chat with other servants and (more relevantly to the context of the present study) with the members of the homes in which she works. Most such servants in fact take a keen interest in the lives of their mistresses and on any working morning can be heard offering and accepting loud and free advice on sundry matters.

At this point, it may be worthwhile to describe briefly the household of a typical employer, since this is where the domestic servant spends the greater part of her day and where, according to our hypothesis, she imbibes her more modern outlook towards life. Most of these servants work in middle- or upper-middle-class homes situated in relatively clean and uncrowded localities. The usual such home would certainly possess the two basic luxuries of modern urban life: a refrigerator and a television set. In addition, it may own some means of transportation (not necessarily a car), the children go to English-language private schools and, most influential of all, there is a general (even if often superficial) air of culture, knowledge, and confidence.

The other common form of employment for the South Indian women is home-based, but involves, if anything, even more interaction with the outside community (albeit of a lower socio-economic status) than does domestic service. This home-based form of self-employment exploits the national popularity of South Indian snacks; so a number of the Tamil women in our sample use a part of the small space which makes up their home to fry *dosas* and *vadas* in the afternoons and then hawk these snacks (the market consists mainly of men and children of all regional groups) in the narrow lanes of the colony in the early evenings. While such interaction with their peers may not add much to their level of knowledge and modernization, it does help to increase their self-confidence and ability to deal with strangers. Such self-confidence is also boosted by the knowledge that they are often the main breadwinners in their families. As seen in row 7 of Table 2.3, the Tamil women are much less likely to have husbands with regular jobs than are the North Indian women. This implies that, even if the working women are not the sole earners in their households, the uncertainties inherent in the more irregular or informal jobs of their husbands mean that the women's incomes are often the core, rather than the trimmings of the household economy.

Rows 4 and 5 of Table 2.3 are also interesting. The results for Tamil Nadu suggest that education acts as a break on employment. This tendency has been noted by others (for example, see Singh 1984) and the reason is probably that the women with some education are less willing to take up the kinds of low status jobs which is the most that the city can offer to women of their slight education and low social class. On the other hand, the few women from Uttar Pradesh in our study who do have some education belong to a particularly innovative group to begin with (as they form part of a system of overall greater female illiteracy) and therefore they are (*a*) more likely to be innovative enough to want to work as well and (*b*) have higher mean levels of education than their educated South Indian counterparts and therefore have access to slightly better occupations.

Finally, I turn to assets. As row 11 of Table 2.3 indicates, these are meagre enough. Anyone with some experience of the Delhi summer can easily appreciate the physical discomfort of the 98 per cent of our respondent households that do not even have a fan to circulate a breeze. But both our regional groups are equally disadvantaged in this regard. The interesting regional differential is in the ownership of a sewing-machine. This appliance is much more likely to belong to a North Indian household, not because of this household's greater wealth but because of the North Indian culture itself, which views the ability to sew as an important qualification in women. This value attached to sewing skills is derived not only from the household savings possible with its use but also because sewing for an income is one of the few respectable occupations that these women can usefully take up, based as it is in the home and requiring contact with an almost exclusively female clientele. On the other hand, seamstress potential has never been an important qualification for the Tamil Nadu women either in their places of origin or in Delhi; their greater freedom to choose from a range of possible occupations makes sewing just one of several possibilities.

This leaves us with regional differentials in our respondent women's pre-marital backgrounds. And, perhaps not too surprisingly, these differentials are of the same kind as the regional differences in our respondent women themselves. To put it succinctly, on the whole it appears that the South Indian woman's parental home is likely to be much more backward economically and yet much more innovative or modern socio-culturally than the Uttar Pradesh woman's home. For example, the Tamil woman's father is (a) more likely to be (have been) an agricultural labourer than a farmer while the reverse is true of the North Indian woman; and (b) has much fewer assets in terms of land and property than the North Indian father. But at the same time, educational levels of our Tamil respondent's fathers (and even of their mothers) are appreciably higher than those of the Uttar Pradesh women's parents; our Tamil women have had fewer siblings, and a smaller proportion of them have died. So on the whole, the pattern of regional differences does not seem to have been disturbed over the last two generations, and over space (that is, in the move from the village to the city).

2.4. The Child Described

We have a lot to say about child births and child deaths in the following chapters. But what about the period in between? In Chapters 5 and 6 we only consider those aspects of this intervening period which are relevant to health and mortality and therefore consider in depth matters such as immunization, diet, and health care. Here we would like to concentrate on other aspects of the child's upbringing and use this not just to point out cultural variation in such upbringing but also to bring out some of the policy implications of these variations.

We begin with the child's social life. In a sense this is an unnecessary aspect to consider because of the intensely social nature of the everyday life of the slum child, whatever its region of origin. First of all, for strongly cultural reasons (and in our present context, for reasons of limited physical space as well) there is very little separation of the child's world from the adult's world. This continuous interaction between different generations in the South Asian milieu has been noted by several anthropologists and can be interpreted as an advantage (through the feeling of security and sense of active belonging that it imparts) or a disadvantage (via the absence of a private transitional phase between babyhood and adulthood) for children, depending on one's own perspectives in this matter. The important point is that a majority of our households did not feel a need to plan any special social activities for their children. Our low figure of a little over one outing per child over the six-month longitudinal study must not be taken to mean that the children were lonely: first, they had enough of a social and community life within the slum itself, and secondly, this did not mean that the parents enjoyed an active social life leaving the children behind; neither generation perceived a need for what our questionnaire dubiously called 'social outings'.

At the same time it must be stressed that the same practical reason, that is poverty, which often meant that parents and children had no escape from each other, sometimes also worked in exactly the opposite way. By remaining away from home for long hours during the day, a lot of the working mothers left their children to their own devices and fully 20 per cent of the Tamil children of working mothers were coded 'No-one' for a question on who looked after them during the day. However, this forced separation between parents and children must be clearly distinguished from any conscious attempt to exclude the child from the adult world. Not only were the children participating prematurely in the adult world of employment and housekeeping, they also often precociously listened wide-eyed to and sometimes even joined in on adult conversations on supposedly adult topics such as sex and its ramifications (including our own detailed enquiries about post-partum abstinence and amenorrhoea!)

Setting aside the fun and games in the child's life, the most striking finding (and also the finding most pregnant with policy implications) is displayed in Table 2.4. This is the general disadvantage faced by the Tamil children in education, contrary to their advantages in survival chances which come out in later chapters. This is in sharp contrast to the regional pattern of education in the two states of origin as well as among our women respondents, and it is what leads to the abrupt reversal of ranks found, for example, in the fact that in our sample households, in the age-group 20–39 years, 8 per cent of the women from Uttar Pradesh and 15 per cent of those from Tamil Nadu were literate, while in the younger (and supposedly more advanced) age-group

Table 2.4. % of children under 12 who attend school

Age-group of children	Uttar Pradesh (N=700)		Tamil Nadu (N=478)	
	Boys	Girls	Boys	Girls
5–9	81	68	74	50
10–11	96	84	68	33

of 10–19 years the corresponding figures are 70 per cent and 30 per cent. That is, the households from northern India are taking much greater advantage of the educational facilities available. In later chapters so much time is spent extolling the demographically 'superior' position of our South Indian sample, that it is necessary to discuss their apparent retrogression in the matter of children's education a little more fully, especially because of the recent world-wide concern about the quality of life being as important an indicator of welfare as its quantity or duration.

Tables 2.5 and 2.6 suggest that most of this observed Tamil disadvantage in schooling can be attributed to practical as opposed to intrinsic or cultural factors. This is fortunate because practical issues are so much more amenable to change than deeply entrenched values and attitudes. Moreover, it appears that it is precisely because the South Indian households are so much more open to innovation and notions of female autonomy (both of

Table 2.5. % of children going to school according to selected maternal characteristics

	Uttar Pradesh (N=700)				Tamil Nadu (N=478)			
	Age Group				Age group			
	5–9		10–11		5–9		10–11	
	Boy	Girls	Boys	Girls	Boys	Girls	Boys	Girls
Maternal Education								
None	80	68	96	82	75	48	64	27
Some	92	71	100	100	73	55	80	50
Maternal Occupation								
None	80	67	96	85	80	48	73	44
Some	93	88	100	77	71	51	66	30

which tend to reduce birth- and death-rates according to our study's hypotheses) that the children suffer in this matter of exposure to education.

First, there is the sex differential in the proportions of children going to school. Table 2.4 shows that (notwithstanding the absence of a clear discrimination against girls in the matters of nutrition and health care) boys from Tamil Nadu are much more likely to receive some schooling than girls and to receive schooling beyond a certain age than are girls. But while overall school-attendance levels are higher for the children from Uttar Pradesh, here too the sex differential operates. For the Tamil group, the greatest sex divergence occurs in the 10–12 year age-group. Girls are progressively more likely to be removed from school than are boys. But 10–12 years of age is still very young and Table 2.4 becomes even more pessimistic about the welfare of girls when looked at in conjunction with Tables 2.5 and 2.6. These girls in the age-group of 10–12 years are most likely to be removed from school if their mothers work or have several children. In both cases the motivation is clear: the girls are kept at home not because school is an unattractive proposition but because there are now new demands on their time and labour. Table 2.6 makes this plain enough: fully 37 per cent of the non-school-going girls aged 10–12 years from the South Indian sample either go out to work or are needed at home. And this is still the pre-adolescent stage; with rising age, these responsibilities and duties can only increase.

But while the Tamil girl seems to be so badly hampered in her educational progress, it is not all roses for her brothers either. Indeed, even where schooling is concerned, the Tamil households continue to show a relatively greater equality in their treatment of boys and girls than do their North Indian counterparts: as many as 25 per cent of the non-school-going boys aged 10–11 years are employed and even in the 5–9 year age-group, 9 per cent of them are needed to help out at home. This is less than the 19 per cent of girls so needed, but a high figure nevertheless when contrasted with the Uttar Pradesh sample, where girls can be withdrawn from school because they are needed at home but this excuse never applies to the boys. Finally, for both groups financial constraints appear to be a much more valid reason for not sending girls to school than for the boys.

In Table 2.6, there is also an interesting cultural response. In

Table 2.6. Reasons for children's non-attendance at school (%)

	Uttar Pradesh				Tamil Nadu			
	Age-group				Age-group			
	5–9		10–11		5–9		10–11	
	Boy	Girls	Boys	Girls	Boys	Girls	Boys	Girls
Child employed	n.s.	n.s.	n.s.	n.s.	5	4	25	29
Child needed at home	n.s.	5	n.s.	6	9	19	n.s.	8
Parents cannot afford to send child to school[a]	13	17	20	24	19	21	21	31
School too far from home	n.s.	n.s.	n.s.	12	n.s.	3	n.s.	2

Note. Since the table gives only the main reasons for non-attendance, where numbers were very low they have been considered not significant, 'n.s.'.

[a] Although schooling is free in principle the 'cannot afford' category turned out to reflect an important parental perception of the costs of schooling, either direct or indirect.

a high percentage of cases, North Indian girls aged 10–12 years are not sent to school because the school is considered to be 'too far'. However, given that all the local Hindi-medium schools (which is where the North Indian children study) are within easy walking distance of the home, the space to be traversed between the home and the school is psychological rather than physical and fits in well with our recorded (in later chapters) greater protectiveness from the outer world towards daughters in the Uttar Pradesh homes. On the other hand, this reason of the school being too far is made much less frequently for the Tamil girls (and for the boys it is not made at all), even though to attend the Tamil-medium secondary school they do have to travel a fair distance into the heart of the city.

A few further points about children's schooling are of interest.

First, as expected, Table 2.5 does indicate that educated mothers are more likely to send their children to school than are uneducated mothers. But we also find that such openness to innovation is greater in our Tamil households in general, including those in which the women are uneducated. This might seem to contradict the last few paragraphs at first sight, but only until one looks at some further details about school-going children. Our data suggest that the decision not to send children to school is almost always taken for purely practical (and mainly economic) reasons; but once children are sent to school, the South Indian households are much more conscious of the quality of the education they choose. For example, the Tamil children are much more likely than those from Uttar Pradesh households to be going to a private school rather than a government-run free school, and (even more importantly) are also much more likely to be going to an English-medium rather than a vernacular (that is, Hindi for the North Indians and Tamil for the South Indians) school. This is especially so if this English-speaking school also happens to be run by Christian missionaries (this is the ultimate status symbol). In general we found that the more the demands on parental energy and (especially) money made by such private schools, the greater was the parental pride in the excellent education that their wards were receiving.

This then is the world of our sample child. On the whole the South Asian culture tends to overwhelm regional variations, so that the similarities between the two groups are greater than the differences. These include the freedom to roam around the narrow lanes of the slum at will (but only until puberty for the North Indian girls), the freedom to interact with adults often on equal terms, and the pressure to shoulder household and economic responsibilities at a relatively early age (especially if the child happens to be Tamil and female). There are a few other interesting regional differences in the level of physical seclusion with approaching adolescence but we discuss these in other chapters because they have a wider relevance. For example, there is the finding that the older North Indian girls are much less likely to use the public taps and toilets than their brothers and than the South Indian girls; a finding with important implications for health and hygiene and therefore brought up more than once in this report.

2.5. Discussion

This chapter has tried to people the environment of the field study. While the primary focus has been on the cultural differences in the two study populations, we hope we have also been able to demonstrate the basic similarities in their social and economic circumstances. These similarities make the differentials in demographic behaviour which emerge in later chapters even more interesting, because they suggest a strong and independent influence of cultural background.

Finally, we shall draw attention to a few points about modernization. We have much to say on women's status and autonomy later, especially in Chapter 3. Here we want to mention one more aspect of the generally more modern outlook of our South Indian households. The central recognition in this outlook is that the woman's time is important, which is shown by the fact that about 95 per cent of our Tamil households use the more expensive gas or kerosene for cooking rather than the more time-consuming and inconvenient fuels such as coal or firewood, while this figure is 82 per cent for the Uttar Pradesh households, even though the latter group is economically better off than the former. Similarly, a small, but significant, proportion of the men in Tamil households help with housework, compared to none of the North Indian men, who do, however, do some shopping for food, but then this once again deprives the women of an enjoyable extra-household activity. Similarly, the boys in the South Indian households help out more (the contribution of girls is high in both groups, but the sex differential is greater for the North Indian families).

However, just like demographic behaviour, this greater modernization is again independent of regional differences in socio-economic status. At the same time, Section 2.4 urges caution in the interpretation of these differentials in women's autonomy and household modernity. Given the low resource base from which our households operate, these apparently positive features of the South Indian culture may be having an adverse impact on at least one group of household members, the children, perhaps not in terms of their survival itself but certainly in the quality of their day-to-day life.

3

The Status of Women

THIS chapter elaborates on the concept of the 'status of women', a term that crops up repeatedly in this book, and whose hypothesized relationship with cultural identity and demographic behaviour we seek to develop. We use a North India–South India classification to divide women into two relatively homogeneous cultural groups. We already know that there are important cultural differences in the northern and southern regions of India and that there are significant differences in demographic indices in the two regions. We also know from secondary data that there are regional differences in some indicators of the status of women, such as education, employment, and age at marriage. But we could do with better evidence on cultural differentials in status-of-women indicators which are more directly related to demographic behaviour, and the following sections therefore use primary data as well as secondary sources to demonstrate such differentials.

3.1. The Status of Women Defined

Before demonstrating a cultural difference in the status of women, the question of the very meaning of the term 'status of women' needs to be settled. With increasing academic and lay interest in gender as distinct from class issues, the term has become extremely value-laden rather than purely descriptive. Hence for the present purposes, where only those aspects of women's position relevant to demographic behaviour are the focus, perhaps it would be best to jettison the term altogether and refer to something more neutral such as the 'role of women' or the 'position of women' or even something as direct as the 'knowledge, attitudes, and practices of women in the areas of fertility and health'. In this way we will avoid getting into the highly important but, in the present context, relatively marginal issue of what constitutes a high or low status of women. The difficulties in resolving such an issue are well illustrated by the controversy in the literature about the relationship between purdah or female seclusion and female status (for a helpful attempt to bring the two sides in this debate together, see Mason 1984).

However, old habits die hard, and undoubtedly the term 'status of women' will creep into the following paragraphs several times. But it should be noted that such use does not imply any kind of objective or even subjective ranking in the present study. For example, as Sharma (1980a) has stressed, in many high status groups, women are proud of their economic and non-economic dependence on men. The less the woman is in control of her own life, the greater the prestige she may enjoy. This is partly why several writers have noted a tendency for women in North India to withdraw from the labour-force as soon as household economic conditions allow.

It would thus be unfortunately naïve to equate women's perceptions of happiness or satisfaction with our demographically relevant rankings based on indicators such as independence and exposure. To cite Mandelbaum's (1988b) reference to an English-woman writing of the life of upper-class Muslim women in North India in the nineteenth century, she repeatedly urged 'her English readers not to judge Indian Muslim customs by the standards of their own society, or to gauge a Muslim woman's unhappiness by how an Englishwoman might feel if she were placed in purdah'.

But to end such digression, let us return to the subject of women's position and demographic behaviour. Our findings suggest that three separate but interdependent components of women's position are especially relevant. These are:

(a) the extent of exposure to the outside world;
(b) the extent of interaction with the outside world, and in particular, the extent of economic interaction; and
(c) the level of autonomy in decision-making within and outside the household.

It should be stressed that we are concerned here with absolute levels of women's position on the above variables, not necessarily their levels relative to the men in their households although, admittedly, the two are usually strongly connected. But theoretically it is possible to conceive of a situation where women in a certain group *A* have as much exposure and interaction with the outside world as the men in their group but (overall levels of exposure and interaction being very low in this group) nevertheless have lower absolute values on these indicators than women in group *B*, whose men are, however, even more advanced than the women.ʼ According to our hypothesis, levels of fertility and mortality will be lower in group *B* although levels of gender inequality on our relevant variables are greater. That is, we are comparing the status of women relative to other women. In the case of autonomy in decision-making, however, since someone has to make the decisions on most matters (though not necessarily on all matters; a tendency to take things as they come is not really as uncommon as might be expected by the typical motivated and non-fatalistic individual), a lower level of female autonomy in decision-making does imply a greater inequality with males.[1]

Perhaps all the above sounds rather faint-hearted and tolerant of prevailing gender inequalities. However, the intention is quite the contrary. The main point being made is that however advanced and independent the men in a community are, there is little hope for desirable changes in demographic behaviour if the women do not grow as well (the negative effect of gender inequality on other aspects of women's welfare is not considered here).

3.2. Some Predictors of the Status of Women

While the present field study iṣ concerned with cultural background as a determinant of the status of women defined as in the last section, this status can conceivably be affected by other non-cultural factors as well. As discussed later on, two of the most powerful such factors appear to be education and employment. But setting these aside for a moment to consider cultural influences, here again one can consider, as the literature has done in the Indian North–South context, a range of influences. For instance, religion, or patriarchal kinship structure, or a history of foreign invasions, can be associated with norms governing women's rankings on our indicators. And if one goes far enough back in time, one can often find economic rationales for the development of these norms and institutions governing women's behaviour.

However, such norms and institutions may be defined as

cultural in the sense that they tend to be accepted by groups with other things in common (such as language or region) than economic circumstances and, secondly, to be slower to change than the economic circumstances which led to their development in the first place. The cultural roots of differences in women's status therefore can be of several different kinds, depending on the culture being studied. But since demographic behaviour is believed to be affected by the status of women rather than by the cultural pattern which gives rise to such status, our hypothesis of the association between the status of women and demographic behaviour can be applied to a variety of cultural groups. What we need are some direct indicators of the position of women as defined in terms of exposure, interaction and autonomy.

But before moving to such direct indicators, since we are using a North India–South India comparison to illustrate our hypothesis, it may be worthwhile to consider in a little more detail the possible cultural attributes that conceivably lead to North–South differences in the position of women. Our survey of the literature and the findings from the field study suggest that in such a North–South comparison, the two most important cultural influences are (*a*) marriage and kinship patterns, and (*b*) the potential for female employment. The next section describes regional differences in these two likely cultural determinants of the status of women.

3.3. Kinship, Marriage, and Women's Economic Roles

In this Section I outline the main features of kinship rules, marriage patterns, and women's economic position that distinguish the North from the South of India. There are several variations within regions, of course, and there has also been change (see, for example, Caldwell, Reddy, and Caldwell 1983); here I focus more on broad intra-regional similarities in behaviour, both actual and idealized. In most of the northern and southern parts of the country, the family is predominantly patrilineal, patrilocal, and patriarchal. But because of major differences in marriage practices between the two regions, this family structure ends up having profoundly different implications for the day-to-day as well as long-term functioning and status of its members, especially its women.

These marriage practices have been discussed in several places (see especially the intricate detail provided by Karve 1965) and here I will describe only those essential features which I believe have a bearing on the status of women in ways relevant to demographic behaviour. On the whole the northern kinship system is characterized by a principle of expansion and the incorporation of outsiders as wives into the family; while the South represents the principle of immediate exchange and a policy of consolidation of existing kin networks. These differences probably reflect ancient differences in the economy of the two regions, the northern kind of kinship pattern being associated with a primarily pastoral economy and therefore depending on external alliances and the incorporation of outsiders for its strength, while the southern pattern more closely approximates what one would expect in an agricultural economy, whose strength lies in the coming closer of already-related kin alliances (see also McDonald 1985).

In actual practice, what these differing goals of marriage involve is that in the North, a village is an exogamous unit for the purposes of marriage, so that in effect all people belonging to the same caste in the same village behave as if they had a common ancestor. There is also a taboo on marriage with near relations or in the family of the mother, the mother's sister, or the father's sister. Therefore, if a daughter is given in marriage into a particular family in a particular village, another daughter cannot enter the same family or village in the same or the next two generations at least. This results in the new bride being thrown into a situation where not a single face is familiar. Physically, she is completely cut off from her natal kin (except in a very formal institutionalized way) and emotionally too she is expected to integrate completely into her husband's household.

Besides decreeing village exogamy, North Indian society also frowns upon the exchange of daughters between families or villages. And given that the giver of the bride is supposed to be inferior in status to the receiver, this means that a family that has given a daughter in marriage to another family can never hope to equalize the relationship by receiving a bride from the groom's household in turn. This one-way relationship is characterized by a one-way flow of resources between two groups related by marriage, carried to its extreme in the relatives of the bride refusing to accept even a glass of water in the son-in-law's home and sometimes even his village.

Such formal relations between two groups related by marriage extend in the first few years of marriage (that is, until she has borne the son to extend the lineage) to relations between the bride and her husband's kin group as well. In fact, all over North India there is a sharp distinction drawn between the daughters of a village and its daughters-in-law: 'the entire social world of many village women [in North India] consists of these two contrasting venues, the place where she is the constrained daughter-in-law and the wonderfully freer home in which she is the beloved daughter' (Mandelbaum 1988b). This distinction applies to the freedoms given to women in the home as well as those outside. The latter distinction operates on the principle that in a system of village exogamy in marriage, the daughter of a household is a daughter of the village itself, that is, she is like a sister to the other men in the village and they are thus duty-bound to protect her, not assault her.

The South Indian marriage and kinship system is best described by contrast with the North. The South allows intra-kin marriages (especially between cross-cousins) and marriages within a village. There is usually a give and take of girls between two related groups so that marriages do not acquire the kind of hypergamous character that they do in the North. Most significantly, the girl usually marries among people she has known since childhood who have other kinds of interactions with her parental family besides those arising out of her marriage. As a consequence, not only is she more free to be herself in her new home, she is also much more able to retain the contact with and support of her natal kin. The distinction is well captured in Karve's fascinating account (1965) of the great regional differentials in nomenclature to define relationships between different household members; in the North this system of nomenclature is very clear in distinguishing between women related by birth and by marriage, whereas in the southern states the same word is often used to identify women from both categories.

With respect to women's economic roles, a few clarifications are necessary in the way in which these are defined for the North–South comparison to become more meaningful. In the first place, one needs to distinguish between actual economic activity by women and the potential for economic activity by women. The two are not identical because behaviour is often dictated not by what one does but what one can do. To cite Watkins (1986) in the longitudinal context of the European fertility transition, 'the new ways of making a living that were adopted by some surely expanded the horizons of the possible for others'. By this argument, in a situation where there are opportunities for women's participation in the labour-force and where the involvement of women in such activities is not frowned upon, one would expect to find fewer differentials in behaviour (especially demographic behaviour) between women who are employed and those who are not, in contrast to a situation where women's labour-force participation rates are low because there is less scope for them. Therefore the community or aggregate level comparison is as important an indicator of the effects of women's economic roles as analyses which focus on the individual woman's economic independence. Cain (1984) has made a similar point while discussing the general question of women's status and fertility.

The second distinction is between economic activity as defined by the individuals directly involved and economic activity as defined by the social scientist who tries to place an objective monetary value on each activity that the woman performs. I would argue that, from the standpoint of women's position, the perceptions of women and their larger kin groups are more important than the reality. For example, it makes little sense to fault census estimates of levels of female labour-force participation rates on the ground that they leave out the economic value of women's household maintenance and other non-paid work. The household itself does not count such work as economically valuable (even when it does not suggest that the woman who does only such work is a lady of leisure) and accordingly places a lower economic value on such a woman herself—a process fraught with several distressing consequences for the family as a whole. The answer would lie in either changing household perceptions about the value of women's work or increasing the opportunities for them to be involved in activities which are already perceived as economically valuable; the latter course would probably be less herculean.

In any case, using secondary information on the actual labour-force participation of women as an indicator of both the opportunities for such participation and household perceptions of their economic roles, Table 3.1 finds a very clear difference between the two regions we are concerned with. The sources of these differentials are arguable and interrelated: physical land conditions which facilitate women's involvement (such as rice being the major crop); a large concern with women's chastity and men's honour; a history of invasions from outside which have led to a whole culture of wanting to protect women from the outside eye; or ingrained notions about gender inequalities in abilities. The net result of any or all of these factors is that women in North India are (*a*) less likely to be doing work that is perceived as economically valuable and (*b*) even when they do work, less likely to be involved in waged activities, that is, activities which involve interaction with the outside world, especially the world of men. This is why, in the rural areas, we have a larger proportion of female workers in Uttar Pradesh being cultivators (that is, working their own land), compared to Tamil Nadu where agricultural labour (that is, working for wages on another person's land) is the main source of employment for women workers. And in our urban study, while the South Indian women worked mainly as domestic servants or as petty entrepreneurs hawking home-made snacks in the lanes of the slum, the Uttar Pradesh women (when they worked at all) were primarily involved in activities which centred around traditional home-based feminine skills, such as sewing for an exclusively female clientele. In fact there was an interesting regional differential in the household ownership of a sewing-machine in the study, the appliance being present in 22 per cent of the Uttar

Table 3.1. Women's participation in the labour-force: Rural areas

	Uttar Pradesh	Tamil Nadu
% of women in the labour-force (main workers only)	5	22
% of female main workers that are cultivators	48	23
% of female main workers that are agricultural labourers	35	53

Source: Registrar General of India (1987), *Analysis of the Work Force in India*, Government of India, New Delhi.

Pradesh homes and only 8 per cent of the Tamil homes. This was due not to the former group's greater wealth, but because the North Indian culture tends to view sewing for an income as one of the few respectable occupations that women can take up.

3.4. Direct Measures of the Status of Women

The above regional pattern of marriage practices and women's employment could plausibly lead to regional differences in our indicators of the position of women. But what is the empirical evidence on this? To begin with, it is well known that there is a strong tradition of purdah or female seclusion in much of North India. This term refers to the constraints placed on women's interaction with the outside world in general and the outside world of men in particular. Its origins are debated and probably include a mix of influences: marriage and kinship patterns that place the young married woman in a completely alien environment, a history of invasions from outside and a consequent culture of the protection of women by confinement indoors, an Islamic influence, agricultural practices which have less use for female labour. (On the role of such historical economic factors, see Boserup 1970; Mencher 1978.) But whatever its origins, the result today is that women in North India are much more likely to observe the norms of seclusion that those in the South.

In its narrowest sense, purdah refers to the full or partial veiling of married women in the presence of males, within and outside the home among Hindus and only in the presence of strangers among Muslims. And, as documented by Jejeebhoy (1981), even in this narrow sense, there are strong cultural differentials in this practice. For example, it is practised by about 45 per cent of women in Uttar Pradesh, but only 5 per cent of those in Tamil Nadu. However, the real effects and ramifications of female seclusion are much wider. For example, in our study area purdah saw its most relevant expression in the differential use of space by women in the two groups. In general, seclusion norms and controls on mobility effectively cut women off from many spheres of knowledge, interaction, and activity. For the North Indian women, the observance of seclusion norms translated into their avoidance of the outdoors when there were men, especially unknown men, around. Therefore, it was only when the men in the colony had left home for the day that the women gathered outside in small groups to catch up on each other's lives, discuss the latest scandals, and attend to the myriad tasks that a labour-intensive and financially tight domestic economy demands. And as the sun set to the sounds of returning husbands and other men, they again disappeared into the smoke of their indoor stoves. Things were quite different in the South Indian streets. These were readily identifiable by the continued presence of women in the evenings. Indeed, the tired and hungry men from all regions presented these women with an avid market for their snacks and other knick-knacks.

Children, however, continued unrestrained whatever the time of day. As described in the last chapter, there was no attempt to keep children out of adult lives and so the sounds of their play permeated the air as much in the dusk as in the afternoon sun. But here again we need to make a cultural distinction—young children of all regional groups may roam freely, but adolescent and even pre-adolescent girls from the North Indian households were almost as secluded as their mothers and not to be seen socializing in the presence of men. As other chapters bring out, this kind of seclusion extends to other areas of life such as medical care, schooling, and use of public services in general.

In Tables 3.2 and 3.3 our study tries to look at more direct indicators of female exposure, interaction and autonomy, and finds that the expected North–South differential does indeed exist. For every indicator of female position, the Tamil women have values which imply higher levels of exposure and interaction with the outside world and a greater control over decision-making. Some of these regional differences become even more remarkable when one looks at them in conjunction with each other. For example, it is the Tamil women who are much more likely to be employed outside the home and yet it is also the Tamil women who seem to find more time to watch television and to interact with friends both within and outside the colony (in spite of the long hours that their employment usually entails). This finding says a lot about (*a*) their greater willingness and desire to interact with the world outside their homes, and (*b*) the greater control which they have over their lives to be able to indulge such desires. The much stronger tradition of female seclusion in our North Indian sample has already been discussed, but it is not clear

Table 3.2. Regional differences in the position of women with respect to exposure to and interaction with the outside world (%)

| Indicator of women's position | Uttar Pradesh (N=642) | | | | Tamil Nadu (N=578) | | | |
| | Age-group | | | | Age-group | | | |
	15–29	30–49	50 +	All ages	15–29	30–49	50 +	All ages
1. Have some education	17	7	0	11	29	21	4	23
2. Are gainfully employed	3	8	13	6	59	75	52	65
3. Watch television regularly	15	10	4	12	20	16	11	18
4. Listen to the radio regularly	21	14	4	17	29	21	11	24
5. Meet friends in the colony regularly	7	7	4	7	23	25	17	23
6. Meet friends outside the colony regularly	2	2	0	2	7	7	11	7
7. Chat with neighbours regularly	18	16	9	17	16	13	5	14
8. Meet their parents regularly	17	8	4	12	45	29	7	35
9. Go out with their husbands regularly	1	1	0	1	13	4	2	8
10. Never go out with their husbands	21	19	17	20	19	34	48	28

whether it is (*a*) or (*b*) above which is largely responsible. The truth is probably that both exist and strengthen each other; that is, in the Uttar Pradesh women, the lesser ability to interact freely with groups outside the formal kinship or neighbourhood structure leads to a lesser knowledge and therefore interest in this psychologically distant outside world and the latter in turn makes it easier for the household to exert greater control on their movements.

There are a few more interesting anomalies in Table 3.2. The one variable on which the women from Uttar Pradesh score higher than their Tamil Nadu counterparts is that described in row 7: the percentages of women who regularly chat with their neighbours. We have already discussed the tendency for urban migrants to cluster residentially in kinship and regional groups, so what this variable really means is that the North Indian women spend a lot of time with their peer groups, in terms of caste and region of origin. In addition it must be added that such interaction with neighbours is almost exclusively interaction with female neighbours so that the world of men outside their immediate homes is wellnigh closed to them. (Indeed, row 9 suggests that their level of informal interaction with the men in their households is rather restricted as well. For example, Madan (1965) describes how, among the Kashmiri Brahmins, the wife is called 'the parrot of the pillow' because she is free to talk to her husband only at night.) Moreover, when the neighbours belong to their kinship group, these are almost always women from their husband's groups that they are exposed to. The general practice of village exogamy in marriage and a somewhat formal subsequent relationship with the natal kin explains row 8 of Table 3.2, where the Tamil women appear to have much greater access to contact with and the support of their parental homes.[2]

This easier access to her parental home probably also serves to increase the South Indian woman's access to resources in her marital home. In only two of the 17 villages in Kerala and Tamil Nadu (both southern states) where Mencher (1989) studied women agricultural labourers did more than 50 per cent of these women hand over their earnings to their husbands. In most households, on the contrary, the men handed their wages to their wives after keeping what they needed for personal expenses. Mencher attributes this control to the South Indian kinship system whereby women are, in the case of Kerala, more free to return to their natal homes and, in the case of Tamil Nadu, either married to relatives or often at least to someone in the same village and sometimes even the same or adjacent street. This is unlike the situation in much of northern India where 'women marry strangers or have to leave their natal village on marriage' (Mencher, 1989).

Then there are the apparently contradictory results in rows 9 and 10 of Table 3.2. Not only are the proportions of women who go out regularly with their husbands much higher for the Tamil Nadu women than for those from Uttar Pradesh, the proportions are similarly much higher also for women who do not go out at all with their husbands. This kind of contradiction caused much confusion in our earlier attempts to construct an index of women's status and forcefully illustrates the need for culture-specific models for defining the position of women. On further analysis of the data and qualitative follow-up of cases it emerged that several of the Tamil women who had very little informal interaction with their husbands were not actually withdrawn wallflowers. On the contrary, their great economic and social importance in managing their households (often single-handedly for all practical purposes) meant that it was the women who did not have the time or inclination to treat their husbands as their equals rather than the other way around.

Finally, we return for a moment to Table 3.3. For both regions there is a very clear increase in household autonomy with age, although at the oldest ages the Tamil women seem to prefer to abdicate some of their responsibilities. The 30–49 year age-group seems to be the one with greatest autonomy and power. This is in line with all anthropological studies of the household in India, especially northern India, where the young wife is seen to be of no consequence until she has demonstrated her worth and loyalty to the household by bearing the necessary sons, of course, but also by integrating completely into her husband's kinship group. Therefore the lowest autonomy levels in Table 3.3 are seen for women aged 15–29 years belonging to the Uttar Pradesh group. But this is also the age-range of women during which fertility and child deaths are most likely to occur, so the consequences of the women's position–demographic behaviour relationship are even more drastic than they would have been had the overall low levels of household autonomy among the Uttar Pradesh women been

Table 3.3. Regional differences in the position of women with respect to autonomy in decision-making (%)

Near total responsibility for	Uttar Pradesh (N=642)				Tamil Nadu (N=578)			
	Age-group				Age-group			
	15–29	30–49	5 0 +	All ages	15–29	30–49	5 0 +	All ages
1. Shopping for food in the market	6	7	13	7	53	55	48	53
2. Deciding on food expenditure	22	35	52	29	54	70	66	62
3. Deciding what to cook	60	71	61	65	68	76	57	70
4. Food distribution at meal-times	70	76	52	72	77	81	70	78
5. Deciding on non-food expenditure	18	26	48	23	35	58	55	47
6. Deciding on a sick child's treatment	27	30	52	29	53	67	61	60

more evenly distributed across women of different ages. Indeed, it is not at all necessary that the low autonomy levels of women of reproductive age reflect correspondingly high autonomy of men in the day-to-day running of the home; what they often indicate is that domestic power resides in the older woman, who is also free to move around outside the home. In this sense, our autonomy indicators comment on the status of relatively young married women *vis-à-vis* other household members, not all of them male.

So Tables 3.2 and 3.3 suggest that the South Indian women are more exposed to the outside world, be it through the mass media, the employer, the shopkeeper, or the local doctor. But the South Indian women are also much more likely than their northern counterparts to be educated, however slightly, and gainfully employed. And both education and employment are directly associated with greater access to and interaction with the extra-household environment. Of course, the higher levels of female literacy and occupation in South India have their origins in a culture which has encouraged these pursuits, but is the Tamil advantage in rows 3 onwards of Table 3.2 and all rows of Table 3.3 only an inevitable consequence of this education and/or employment? We do not think so. To illustrate, Table 3.4 examines educational differences in these indicators of the status of women.[3] As in the case of educational influences on fertility and mortality (discussed in later chapters), three points stand out:

1. Both education and employment appear to be powerful tools for changing women's position in a direction conducive to lower fertility and mortality rates. This is an encouraging finding because it suggests policy interventions that would be more welcome than an assault on factors such as marriage practices.

2. However, educational and occupational differentials in demographically relevant indicators of the status of women are distinctly lower for Tamil Nadu than for Uttar Pradesh. In fact, not only are they lower, they are often in an unexpected direction as well. For example educated Tamil women may take less, not more, of a responsibility for household food expenditure than the uneducated women.

3. More interestingly, within each educational category the Tamil women continue to have higher levels of exposure, inter-action, and autonomy in decision-making than the women from Uttar Pradesh. In fact it is among the uneducated women that

Table 3.4. Educational differences in the position of women (%)

Indicator of women's position	Uttar Pradesh (N=642)			Tamil Nadu (N=578)		
	Level of education			Level of education		
	None	Some	None/some	None	Some	None/some
1. Watch television regularly	12	21	0.6	17	20	0.9
2. Listen to the radio regularly	17	21	0.8	25	21	1.2
3. Have near total responsibility for						
shopping for food in the market	7	14	0.5	54	48	1.1
deciding on food expenditure	29	36	0.8	63	57	1.1
deciding what to cook	65	79	0.8	70	79	0.9
food distribution at meal-times	72	64	1.1	78	82	1.0
deciding on expenditure on food and non-food items	23	39	0.8	46	47	1.0
deciding on a child's treatment	29	50	0.6	60	59	1.0

regional differences in these indicators of the status of women are the greatest, suggesting strongly that it is not education which accounts for the bulk of regional differentials. Indeed cultural background seems to be functioning in the same way as education or a gainful occupation to influence the position of women and through this their fertility and child mortality levels.

To be sure, the cultural factor can in turn be disaggregated into a number of more specific components (as already discussed, we would place paramount among these the drastically different kinship systems in the two regions and the strong differences in the economic roles of women) and also, what constitutes a 'cultural' explanation in short-run analysis may in the long run turn out to be 'economic' (see Basu, Jones, and Schlicht 1987). But our point is that these disaggregated characteristics are so intrinsic to the specific culture of each of the regions considered that attributing our observed regional differences to these characteristics is equivalent to attributing them to their distinct cultural identities.

It does therefore seem to be the case that there are cultural differences in the position of women which persist even after we have controlled for differences in the socio-economic circumstances as well as the external environment of the households from these two cultural backgrounds. But how do differences in the position of women translate into differences in demographic behaviour? The next three chapters have much to say on this question; here one can briefly mention that they work through differences in knowledge, attitudes, and practices in areas related to fertility, health, and mortality. Or, to quote Dyson and Moore (1983), through differences in the ability to 'obtain information and to use it as the basis for making decisions about one's private concerns and those of one's intimates'. This process quite clearly involves two needs—the access to resources (in this case knowledge, information, and services) and the freedom to use these in any way—that are well subsumed under the three broad variables that go to make up our measure of the position of women.

The question of 'prestige' or 'esteem' as an aspect of women's status is irrelevant in this context and may well be the highest in those groups which score lowest on our indicators. But they are of course important from the individual woman's point of view, and

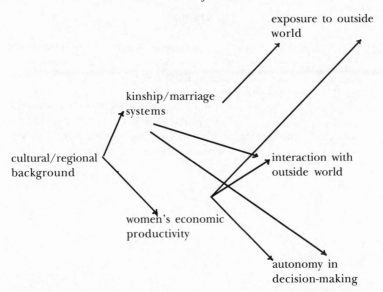

FIG. 3.1. A model of the factors influencing the status of women in North and South India

the determinants of her sense of achievement and happiness are not to be taken lightly (see, for instance, Table 7.1) even if they are derived from what economists call imperfect information.

3.5 Discussion

A formal model of North–South differentials in the status of women in India would therefore resemble that illustrated in Fig. 3.1. Subsequent chapters add to this model, assisting our understanding of the mechanisms involved in its relationships with fertility, childhood mortality, and sex differentials in physical well-being.

NOTES

1. That is, as discussed more fully in Chapters 6 and 7, to understand sex differences in physical welfare, one needs to look at our women's status indicators relative to the men in these cultures.
2. On this point, see also Mandelbaum 1988*b*.
3. Incidentally, the pattern of regional differences in the indicators of the position of women according to the women's occupational status is very similar to that based on whether the women have had any education. Accordingly, a separate table is not presented.

4

Fertility

STUDIES of historical fertility declines, such as in Europe (Coale and Watkins 1986), have repeatedly come upon the importance of geographical location as a determinant of fertility differentials as well as of the process of fertility change. Since regional groups that historically exhibited similar demographic behaviour simultaneously exhibited a range of economic conditions, it appears that economic factors alone cannot explain such geographical similarities in demographic behaviour. More cultural explanations are needed, culture being defined in several ways to include factors such as region, religion and language.

With a similar emphasis on non-economic variables, this chapter examines the regional differential in fertility in India and some of the possible influences on this differential. We already know from secondary data that there are marked fertility differences between the states of Tamil Nadu and Uttar Pradesh (for example see Registrar General of India, 1981*b*, 1983*a*, 1983*b*; and Table 1.1, above) but these can theoretically be attributed to regional differences in the extra-household (particularly governmental) supports for controlled fertility. In the field study which provides the primary data for the present analysis, such supports are common to both groups, micro-economic variations in the demand for children are largely controlled, and yet, in Section 4.1 we find a cultural difference in fertility, the South Indians exhibiting lower levels than the North Indians. Sections 4.2 and 4.3 explore the mechanisms and motivations behind these fertility differences and conclude that (*a*) in spite of important and interesting differences in the proximate determinants of natural fertility, earlier volitional termination of childbearing is the principal means by which marital fertility differences are obtained; and (*b*) such volitional fertility control is greater in the case of respondents from Tamil Nadu because of a greater diffusion of the small family norm itself in these respondents, a

Table 4.1. Regional differentials in cumulative
marital fertility

| | Mean number of children ever born | | | |
| | Present survey | | 1981 census—rural areas | |
Age-group	Uttar Pradesh (N=642)	Tamil Nadu (N=578)	Uttar Pradesh	Tamil Nadu
15–19	0.68	1.10	0.29	0.46
20–24	2.23	1.92	1.27	1.21
25–29	3.69	3.30	2.59	2.29
30–34	4.34	3.67	3.71	3.15
35–39	4.57	4.32	4.61	3.81
40–44	5.48	4.94	5.08	4.00
45–49	5.96	5.03	5.33	4.11
5 0 +	6.78	5.43	5.05	3.84
All ages[a]	3.87	3.43	3.15	2.66

[a] Standardized according to the age distribution of married women in the Uttar Pradesh survey sample

Source: for census data, Registrar General of India (1983), *Census of India 1981, Part II: Special Report and Tables Based on 5 per cent Sample Data* (Series 22 for Uttar Pradesh and Series 20 for Tamil Nadu) Government of India, New Delhi.

diffusion which has been considerably aided by the higher levels of female authority and autonomy in this group. As stated in Chapter 1, the Tamil Nadu–Uttar Pradesh comparison is illustrative; it is predicted that similar results will be obtained in a comparison of any two groups differentiated by the status of women as defined in Chapter 3. Section 4.4 comments on the sex preferences underlying higher fertility in India in general and North India in particular; while Section 4.5 considers the role of the hitherto (perhaps unfairly) neglected partner in reproductive behaviour—the husband.

4.1. Regional Differentials

I begin this section with a comparison of fertility data from the survey with secondary data from the respondents' states of origin. The first striking thing about Tables 4.1 and 4.2 is that, whatever

Table 4.2. Regional differentials in age-specific
marital fertility rates

Age-group	Present survey[a]		1981 census	
	Uttar Pradesh (N=642)	Tamil Nadu (N=578)	Uttar Pradesh	Tamil Nadu
15–19	166.7	268.3	85.0	181.0
20–24	358.3	339.0	201.0	241.0
25–29	348.4	232.0	214.0	194.0
30–34	249.3	137.5	187.0	126.0
35–39	108.7	74.1	138.0	71.0
40–44	32.8	20.8	85.0	29.0
45–49	0.0	0.0	43.0	10.0
5 0 +	0.0	0.0	0.0	0.0
Total marital fertility rate	6321.0	5358.5	4765.0	4260.0

[a] Based on an average of births in the last three years

Source: for census data: Registrar General of India (1988), *Census of India 1981, Fertility in India: An Analysis of 1981 Census Data,* occasional paper no. 13 of 1988, Government of India, New Delhi.

the fertility indicator, our sample groups have considerably higher levels than their sisters in the states of origin. Not only is cumulative fertility higher (Table 4.1), current fertility (Table 4.2) also shows a similar trait, even though our data refer to a later period than the 1981 census from which the secondary figures have been obtained. Does this mean that the move to the city has led to higher fertility in our sample groups? Such an occurrence would be odd and would go against most established theories about the role of migration and urban residence on fertility behaviour. Nor do we have much reason to believe that our study respondents' behaviour is so different from what is expected. Instead, the anomaly seems to stem from two factors:

1. Ours is a selective sample. All its members are migrants of course, but, as discussed in Chapter 1, they are not really a biased group for this reason. The reason they are a biased group is that these households do not represent a random selection of migrants

from Uttar Pradesh or Tamil Nadu. Instead they represent the lowest socio-economic classes in their states of origin, classes which even secondary sources find have above-average fertility levels. For example, the 1979 survey by the Registrar General of India (1981*b*) found that for illiterate rural women in Uttar Pradesh, the total marital fertility rate was 6.7, while for literate women it was 6.4 (the contrast was much sharper in the urban areas); for rural Tamil Nadu, corresponding figures were 4.8 and 4.4. The differences would probably be even sharper if we could take other socio-economic class variables into account.

2. A more important reason for the higher fertility of our sample women as compared to their counterparts in the home state is the greater reliability of our responses. In a sense this is only to be expected, given that the relative ease of accurate data collection is one of the major advantages of micro-level surveys as opposed to a census or large-scale survey. A quick examination of just one possible source of fertility under-reporting confirms this feeling. The sex ratio (males per 1000 females) of all births to our respondents works out to 1150 for the Uttar Pradesh respondents and 1017 for those from Tamil Nadu. The figure for Uttar Pradesh is doubtful enough and the difficulties in recording all dead daughters have already been discussed in an earlier chapter. But our pestering of respondents to provide a complete birth history seems to have yielded more reliable estimates than those from the 1981 census: the sex ratios of children ever born to women in rural Uttar Pradesh and Tamil Nadu in this census were 1171 and 1088 respectively.

To return to regional differentials in fertility in our study, for both cumulative and current fertility, levels are consistently lower for Tamil Nadu than for Uttar Pradesh (Tables 4.1, 4.2, and 4.3). In fact, the differential would be greater if one corrected for the under-reporting of dead daughters in the North Indian sample as just mentioned. While we discuss the possible mechanisms involved in these fertility differences in the next section, the pattern of this fertility differential is worth considering briefly here. To begin with, the difference seems to be greater for current than for cumulative fertility, suggesting that the two groups are reacting differently to their presently similar circumstances. Secondly, in the age-group of 15–19 years, the regional difference in fertility (both cumulative and current) is in a strikingly opposite direction

Table 4.3. % of women with four or more children ever born

Age-group	Uttar Pradesh (N=642)	Tamil Nadu (N=578)
15–29	35.2	21.9
30–49	75.1	63.2
5 0 +	86.9	76.8
All ages[a]	56.1	44.3

[a] Standardized according to the age distribution of married women in the Uttar Pradesh sample.

to that for other age-groups—the Tamil women have marital fertility levels almost twice those of their North Indian counterparts. We feel that one reason for this is the age distribution of women within this age-group: given their higher age at marriage, the Tamil sample in biased towards the older (and therefore theoretically more fecund) ages in this category. Moreover, as we discuss below, the later age at marriage in the Tamil sample is also associated with a faster pace of childbearing in the early years of marriage. Secondly, in Table 4.2 the largest fertility differences are seen in the 30–34 year age-group. This is well within the active childbearing ages, suggesting that volition rather than fecundity is an important cause of fertility differentials.[1]

4.2. Mechanisms

It is not enough merely to demonstrate that cultural or regional background influences achieved fertility levels. The intermediate variables or the biological and behavioural factors which mediate this link between socio-cultural status and fertility need to be identified for a fuller understanding of the relationship, especially if there is also a policy aim of changing fertility behaviour in a specified way. While cultural factors have been proposed as an explanation for regional differences in fertility (see, in particular, Dyson and Moore 1983), there has not been a systematic attempt in the literature to relate cultural practices to the proximate determinants of fertility; the assumption is usually that all the proximate determinants must be affected in some way.

As early as 1956, Davis and Blake drew up a list of eleven intermediate variables through which all other factors must theoretically act to influence fertility levels. More recently, Bon-gaarts (1978, 1982), from an empirical analysis of fertility has narrowed this list to four intermediate factors which affect fertil-ity differentials and trends. These are the age at (first) marriage and proportions never marrying (as proxies of the age at initiation of the risk of pregnancy, and proportions at risk, respectively); contraceptive use; recourse to induced abortion; and the duration of post-partum sterility. In the present study we find it easier to examine regional differentials in the proximate determinants of fertility by grouping these according to the stage of the marital life-cycle during which they take effect. We look at three aspects of the reproductive life of the woman: the initiation of childbearing, the speed of reproduction, and the termination of childbearing. The following pages use field data as well as infor-mation from published sources (primarily the census and large-scale surveys) to identify some of the ways in which cultural background (independently of socio-economic circumstances) affects fertility-related behaviour at these three levels. An attempt is also made to relate the components of cultural background which are hypothesized to be important in the present context—marriage and kinship systems, and the scope for women's parti-cipation in the labour-force—to the proximate determinants of fertility thus identified as relevant.

Furthermore, this section concludes that while there are impor-tant regional differences in some of the proximate determinants of fertility, in particular in the ages at marriage and at the first live birth, final fertility differentials can be explained mainly by differences in one proximate determinant, the parity-specific volitional termination of childbearing. This result is due to the fact that the region with relatively early marriage is also the region in which, for various reasons connected with marriage practices, the gap between effective marriage and the first birth is relatively large. This means that, in the end, differences in natural fertility between the two groups can explain at best a small part of the eventual fertility differential. It is remarkable how similar these cross-sectional results are to those obtained from an analysis of the historical fertility transition in the developed countries. In the latter case too, all evidence suggests that the secular fall in fertility was due almost entirely to the voluntary control of marital fertility, with factors such as nuptiality playing a marginal role at best (Coale and Watkins 1986).

The Initiation of Childbearing

Marriage

Technically, there is no risk of pregnancy before menarche is reached.[2] And in the Indian situation, where there is little sexual activity before marriage, even menarche is only indirectly associated with the start of exposure to childbearing via its relation to the onset of legal cohabitation. Hence, in the Indian (and, indeed, South Asian) context, it is marriage which coincides with the beginning of exposure to the risk of pregnancy, as long as marriage is correctly defined. That is, there is a need to distinguish between the marriage ceremony which formalizes a girl's marital status and the *gauna* ceremony which heralds the start of sexual relations. The former can occur at any age but the latter must typically await puberty. As Table 4.4 demonstrates, the gap between the two events (that is, between rows 1 and 2) is substantial for the Uttar Pradesh women, although there is a trend towards smaller gaps among the younger women, with a gradual convergence of the ages at the two events reaching its peak in the Tamil sample, where marriage occurs well after the onset of menses and where the interval between marriage and cohabitation is often nominal or non-existent. Because of this gap between formal marriage and cohabitation, it makes little sense to talk of the direct effect of cross-sectional differences in the age at marriage or of trends in this variable. In the latter case, as Wyon *et al.* (1966) demonstrate for Punjab, a rising age at marriage has been associated with a falling interval to cohabitation, so that, until the 1960s at least, there was no real change in the age at first exposure to conception.

Therefore, while the age at marriage may be important for fertility in indirect ways[3] (for example, through its curtailment of several freedoms, especially those involving interaction with the outside world), it is the age at *gauna* or effective marriage which is a proximate determinant of fertility in South Asia. And, fortunately for the survey method, this event is much easier to identify and measure than the range of union types which signal exposure to the risk of conception in other parts of the world, a problem that the World Fertility Survey met head-on during its cross-country comparisons. As seen in row 2 of Table 4.4, the Tamil women do have a higher age at effective marriage than the women from

Table 4.4. Regional differentials in the initiation of childbearing

Mean values of indicators	Uttar Pradesh (N=642)				Tamil Nadu (N=578)			
	Age-group				Age-group			
	15–29	30–49	5 0 +	All ages	15–29	30–49	5 0 +	All ages
Age at marriage	9.8	8.2	7.8	8.9	16.4	16.0	15.4	16.1
Age at effective marriage	14.7	15.2	15.7	15.0	16.5	16.2	16.7	16.4
Gap between effective marriage and first live birth, in months	45	54	72	50	22	32	50	29
Age at first live birth	17.8	19.3	21.2	18.7	17.8	18.5	20.5	18.4

Table 4.5. Socio-economic differentials in the mean age
at marriage of currently married women: 1981 census

Socio-economic variable	Mean age at marriage	
	Rural Uttar Pradesh	Rural Tamil Nadu
Education		
Illiterate	15.9	18.2
Literate but below primary	16.4	18.4
Middle but below matric	16.8	18.6
Employment		
Non-workers	16.0	18.4
Workers	15.6	18.3
Cultivators	15.9	18.4
Agricultural labourers	15.2	18.2

Source: Registrar General of India (1988), *Female Age at Marriage: An Analysis of 1981 Census Data,* Government of India, New Delhi.

Uttar Pradesh. Other estimates of the age at marriage (for example, from successive censuses) also show this clear regional differential (although these data sets do not seem to distinguish very clearly between the marriage ceremony and cohabitation).

But why must these North–South differences in the age at effective marriage be culturally determined? It is equally plausible that the differences reflect regional differences in socio-economic factors and have nothing to do with cultural identity as such. Several lines of reasoning can be used to diminish the force of this argument. To begin with, the primary data used here relate to socio-economically very similar groups, both composed of poor slum-dwellers belonging to two distinct cultural backgrounds and with little socio-economic heterogeneity within each group. And yet there is a clear differential in the age at marriage between the two. The role of culture and region becomes even clearer in data from the census, where the age at marriage in the socio-economically more mixed populations of the two states is disaggregated by standard socio-economic indicators (see Table 4.5). Once again, it appears that even in the case of the otherwise powerful variable of education, there is hardly any difference in the mean age at marriage of women until they have gone well beyond middle school. Female employment as an explanatory variable shows a similar pattern. First, there is not much difference in the mean age at marriage for working and non-working women and for women working in various manual occupations; secondly, whatever differential there is, exists in the Uttar Pradesh case, but since this is the region with very low labour-force participation rates, women's employment status cannot be a significant factor depressing the marriage age in North India. Bloom and Reddy (1984) also find in their analysis of India that there are no substantial differences in the timing of marriage by religion, caste, or education. This finding, together with their observation that, on the other hand, studies which use aggregate data for a cross-section of villages or states do find such differences, leads them to conclude (incorrectly, I think) that socio-economic differentials that exist across communities do not exist to the same extent within communities. The final clinching point in the Indian case is that even within similar socio-economic categories, cultural differences in the age at marriage are marked: compare, for example, the agricultural labourers from the two states in the census, with the mean age at marriage for those from Uttar Pradesh being a good three years lower than those from Tamil Nadu (Registrar General of India 1988a).

Casting the net a little wider, Trussell and Reinis (1989) conclude from their study of time trends based on analysis of World Fertility Survey data from 41 countries that (a) the age at marriage is variable across countries for all cohorts and (b) only a few countries show marked time trends in the age at marriage; presumably socio-economic changes have not been negligible in all the others. And going further back in time, the Princeton European Fertility Project was able to demonstrate a striking statistical relation between region and nuptiality, a relation which could not be explained simply by regional differences in economic variables (see Watkins 1986). Moreover, even though there were marked changes over time in the proportions married in all regions, until about 1930 the relative level of nuptiality among the regions of most countries remained unchanged. Therefore, socio-economic differentials can provide at best a partial explanation of regional differentials in the age at marriage. How can cultural factors as defined by kinship rules and women's economic position be a stronger influence in the Indian case? To answer this question, one must of necessity be more descriptive; quantitative relations are difficult to establish or even design for study.

To begin with, we have much anthropological and historical material on the expected role of the new wife in the North Indian system of kinship and marriage. To quote one authority on the subject, 'the women generally occupy the inner rooms . . . a bride should neither be seen too much except when working, nor heard too much . . . generally a woman is so dominated by the affinal kin or by the husband that she rarely makes a positive impression except as a mother' (Karve 1965). On the other hand, 'a woman in the South lives and moves freely in her father-in-law's house. She does not usually have to cover her face in the presence of elder males as she does in the Hindi region, nor is she so cut off from her natal family' (*ibid.*). In other words, the North Indian bride is expected to be substantially more pliant and deferential than her southern counterpart. And if we accept that there is a positive link between age and obstinacy (or difficulties in adjustment, to put it more mildly), one can see that the traditional North Indian household is only being rational in seeking younger girls as brides for its men. Add to this the larger role of marriage in forging new alliances between groups (see also McDonald 1985) rather than cementing existing alliances as happens in the South, and the greater hurry to find brides makes even more sense.

What about the girl's family? Here, the incentives to get the girl married early complement those facing the groom's kin group. For one thing, the needs of the latter mean that the older girl is less in demand as a wife, from which it follows that the costs of getting her married are that much higher. These costs also increase because of an expected negative relationship between an unmarried girl's age and her chastity—naturally, since the period of exposure to temptation increases with time. Further, the negligible economic role of the North Indian woman is a major impediment to her continued presence in the parental home. As Dyson and Moore (1983) point out, this pragmatic consideration can explain at least a part of the desire to see her married soon; if she remains unmarried, not only is she not perceived as contributing to her upkeep, she is not even able to contribute to the growth of the increasing fund needed to meet her marriage expenses.

Conversely, in the southern case, an unmarried daughter's economic worth makes her an asset to the parental family and, just as importantly, makes her welcome in her affinal home even at a relatively late age. The fact that this affinal home is more likely to be known to her and related to her by descent as well only helps to make matters easier of course. But in the context of women's economic roles, it is necessary to make a more general point about the different results obtained by different levels of analysis. For example, if one looked solely at the Uttar Pradesh data in Table 4.5, one might be tempted to conclude that working women tend to marry somewhat earlier than women who do not work. But, as discussed earlier, Uttar Pradesh represents a situation of very low female labour-force participation rates, and the few women who do venture out of the home to work represent a selective group consisting largely of those who are driven to seek work because of their extreme poverty. The connection between women's economic roles and the age at marriage is therefore more appropriately examined in the Tamil Nadu case, where working women (in the lower-level occupations) represent a more random selection of all women. The link in this latter case is virtually non-existent, but one can still say that in areas where large proportions of the women are economically active, the average age at first marriage tends to be higher than in areas where few women enter the labour-force. That is, the correct women's employment variable is represented by the opportunities for female employment rather than the individual need for female employment.[4]

Finally, it should be noted that the above cultural differences are only relative: even the South Indian women can hardly be said to be delaying marriage to a significantly late age by modern Western standards. After all, the kinship structure in the South is also largely patrilineal and patriarchal and in neither regional group is the economic independence of men (which is in any case difficult to define) a serious bar to marriage (see Dixon 1971); the difference between the North and the South of India is more in the matter of specific marriage practices within this common overall structure.

The First Child

Having said so much about the cultural influences on the age at effective marriage (and some of this has also been said by others, including Smith 1983, Dyson and Moore 1983), the question that arises is how reliable is the age at marriage as a measure of the initiation of childbearing and hence subsequent fertility? In the absence of deliberate fertility control, it can be hypothesized that late marriage leads to:

(*a*) a reduction in total duration of fecund exposure to sexual activity because of a shift in the latter to the older and therefore less fecund ages;

(*b*) a smaller fraction of each cohort surviving to marry;

(*c*) an increase in the mean length of generation and hence a fall in the population growth-rate (Coale and Tye 1961); and

(*d*) a temporary shift in period fertility. (*b*), (*c*) and (*d*) are macro-level effects, while (*a*) also refers to the impact of delayed marriage on the fertility of individual women.

But it appears to be the case that these relations between the age at marriage and fertility are clearer when one is looking at a culturally homogeneous group. This is because the effect of age at marriage on natural fertility seems to be heavily modified by the first birth interval. Moreover, there seem to be important cultural variations in the length of this interval, variations which are often enough to completely negate any effect on the age at first live birth across cultures of variations in the age at first marriage. Therefore, in a cross-national or cross-cultural context, one is inclined to agree with Hobcraft (1985) that it may be more useful to tie analyses of fertility to the occurrence of the first birth rather than to entry into a sexual relationship.

The last row of Table 4.4 illustrates this point with my survey data. Whatever the regional differences in the first exposure to intercourse and conception the women in the two groups end up having the first child at uncannily similar ages. This in turn means that the two groups have taken different lengths of time after effective marriage to bear the first live birth. This cultural difference in the length of the first birth interval is also clearly apparent in the larger all-India study conducted by the Registrar General of India (1988*b*): at 47 months for rural Uttar Pradesh and 30 months for rural Tamil Nadu, the gaps between effective marriage and the first birth are very similar to our study findings. To add more general support to the validity of these observations is an analysis by Trussel and Reinis (1989) of World Fertility Survey data from 41 countries, which noted that for each cohort in the countries studied, the mean age at first birth was more

Table 4.6. Age-specific fertility rates of women
in rural areas: 1981 census

Age-group	Region	Married (%)	ASFR[a]	ASMFR[b]
15–19	Uttar Pradesh	68	0.058	0.085
	Tamil Nadu	24	0.044	0.181
20–24	Uttar Pradesh	94	0.195	0.201
	Tamil Nadu	79	0.190	0.241

[a] Age-specific fertility rate: the average number of children born alive during the last year per woman in the given age-group.

[b] Age-specific marital fertility rate: the average number of children born alive during the last year per married woman in the given age-group.

Source: Registrar General of India (1988), *Female Age at Marriage: An Analysis of 1981 Census Data,* Government of India, New Delhi

homogeneous across populations than was the mean age at marriage.

The effects of such differences in the first birth interval are well illustrated in Table 4.6, derived from the 1981 census of India. From the overall population standpoint, the great differences in the proportions married in the 15–19 year age-group hardly lead to any great differences in age-specific fertility rates. The answer can be found in the age-specific marital fertility rates in column 5 of Table 4.6. In fact, even for the 20–24 year old age-group (where the possibly greater adolescent sterility associated with a higher proportion of the Uttar Pradesh married women belonging to the lower end of the age-group range cannot be a major factor), there is not much regional difference in age-specific fertility rates in spite of the regional difference in the proportions married.

Admittedly these regional differences in the first birth interval can conceivably have several non-cultural explanations. These include region selective omission of first births, the effect of adolescent sterility associated with early marriage and region specific use of voluntary birth control between marriage and the first child. However, as discussed in Basu (forthcoming), none of these factors seem to provide an adequate explanation in the present context. In particular, see Table 4.7 on the persistence of the long first birth interval in Uttar Pradesh even among women marrying at ages twenty and above (see also, Chidambaran and Zodegekar 1969). McDonald (1984) who found with World Fertil-

Table 4.7. The first birth interval according to age at
effective marriage

Age at effective marriage	First birth interval (months)	
	Rural Uttar Pradesh	Rural Tamil Nadu
< 18	47	28
18–20	40	31
> 20	47	32
All ages	47	30

Source: Registrar General of India (1988), *Birth Interval Differentials in India, 1984*,
Government of India, New Delhi.

ity Survey data that even for women marrying between the ages
of 21 and 24, the length of the first birth interval ranged from
42 months in Nepal to 17 months in the Philippines.

Table 4.7 also makes the 'catching-up' hypothesis (which ex-
pects late marriers to rush to have the first birth) appear less
tenable because the cultural differences in the first birth interval
are much greater than the differences within a homogeneous
culture according to the age at marriage. This conclusion is
strengthened by the Registrar General of India's (1988*b*) finding
that there are no consistent differences in closed birth intervals
according to the age at marriage in either regional group being
considered here. Of course there may be a 'catching-up' process
involved in a long-term institutional sense, in that societies with
a later age at marriage are those with fewer props supporting a
long first birth interval, but this suggestion is too tautologous to
have any significant implications.

We are forced therefore to seek more 'cultural' explanations for
the regional difference in the gap between effective marriage and
the first birth. The only variable which remains as a possible
determinant of differentials in the first birth interval is exposure
to the risk of conception through exposure to intercourse itself.
This can happen in two ways—through regional differences in the
frequency of intercourse in the first years of marriage, and
regional differences in the periods of prolonged abstinence in
the first years of marriage. Both these factors are important
influences on fecundability in general (see Bongaarts and Potter
1983, and Rindfuss and Morgan 1983, for the postulated relationship between intercourse frequency and fertility; and Chen *et al.*

Fertility

1974, Menken 1979, Bongaarts and Potter 1979, van de Walle 1975, and Cain 1985 for discussions on possible temporary abstinence effects on fertility).

What is the evidence on regional differences in these two exposure related factors in India? This evidence is discussed more fully in Basu (forthcoming) and I will only paraphrase it here. The regional differences in marriage and kinship systems outlined in chapter 3 have two characteristics relevant to the variables of interest. First, the relatively subordinate role of the young wife in North India is associated with more restricted contact between husband and wife in the first few years of marriage. This in turn means that the frequency of intercourse is relatively low during this time, compared to their South Indian counterparts, where even young married women have traditionally experienced a greater ease of interaction with their husbands—the often pre-marital acquaintance between spouses is certainly a factor in this respect (see, for example, Mandelbaum 1988a; Srinivas 1976).

The second feature of North Indian kinship that restricts intercourse in the first years of marriage is the practice of village or territorial exogamy. Having the wife come from another village cuts her off from her parental home, as has been noted by several writers. But the complementary situation has been less commented upon and is important for our present purposes. This is the situation of the wife being completely cut off from her husband every time she visits her natal home. These visits are long and frequent during the first years of marriage and carry with them long and frequent periods of temporary abstinence during these early years (for discussions in the literature on the practice of North Indian brides going to their parents for months at a time, see, among others, Sharma 1980b and Jeffery, Jeffery, and Lyon 1989; however, all these authors are interested in this practice for non-demographic reasons). In contrast, in the South, women's absences from the marital home are less formal and extended and, in any case, the frequent overlapping of marital and natal kin also mean that the physical distance to be traversed during such visits is small.

It seems, therefore, that there is not an automatic connection between early marriage and an early start of childbearing, especially in a cross-cultural setting. In turn, cross-cultural differences in nuptiality may have a less central role in determining overall levels of natural fertility. However, it can still be and probably is the case that early marriage is associated with higher fertility for non-biological reasons to do with differences in knowledge, values and ideas; by increasing the exposure to another world, later marriage undoubtedly leads to changes in fertility desires. More-over, both late marriage and low volitional fertility are the result of a common set of socio-economic influences (Coale 1991).

Where does all this leave us? The main conclusion appears to be that nuptiality itself does not seriously influence regional natural marital fertility rates, though it is undoubtedly partly responsible for age-specific birth-rate differentials. Similarly, the age at first live birth does affect fertility but is not a good explanation for observed regional differentials. Finally, the gap between mar-riage and first birth is not a likely explanation for regional fertility differences, although it strongly affects regional differences in early marital fertility as is discussed more fully below.

The Pace of Childbearing

Once childbearing has begun, further differentials in population growth-rates are possible because different groups have sub-sequent births at different speeds, even if final achieved cumula-tive fertility is similar. In the present context, it is convenient to look at two aspects of the speed of childbearing—the rate of childbearing in the early years of married life and the overall rate at which births occur—because these two aspects are influenced by quite different sets of factors.

Row 1 of Table 4.8 finds the pace of early marital fertility to be considerably higher for Tamil Nadu than for Uttar Pradesh in spite of overall fertility being lower. The mean number of births in the first five years of effective marriage for the Tamil group is about four times that for the Uttar Pradesh women in spite of closed birth intervals being remarkably similar in the two groups (see row 2 of Table 4.8) and suggests that the entire variation in early marital fertility is due to variations in the first birth interval. The regional variation in this factor has already been discussed and the further finding that this variation can in turn lead to such great differences in the vulnerable first years of marriage is a sobering one. One wonders what is implied about the effects on maternal and child health (see, for example, National Academy of

Table 4.8. Regional differentials in the pace of childbearing[a]

| | Uttar Pradesh (N=642) | | | | Tamil Nadu (N=578) | | | |
| | Age-group | | | | Age-group | | | |
	15–29	30–49	50 +	All ages	15–29	30–49	50 +	All ages
Mean number of births in first 5 years of marriage	0.5	0.3	0.3	0.4	2.1	1.7	1.0	1.8
Mean gap between births, in months	30	36	36	33	29	37	42	34
% women currently pregnant	11.2	8.2	0.0	9.4	17.7	3.8	0.0	10.4
Mean duration of breast-feeding of living children, in months	24	26	27	26	18	22	26	20
% women who have ever used birth-control	18.2	40.5	17.4	28.8	47.4	60.7	23.2	50.5
% women who have ever used modern non-terminal birth-control	15.0	9.5	0.0	11.8	33.2	13.8	1.8	22.2
% women currently using modern non-terminal birth-control	4.8	2.3	0.0	3.4	15.9	4.2	0.0	9.5

Sciences 1989) and general well-being, and one can only be relieved that it is the more independent and older Tamil women (in comparison to their Uttar Pradesh counterparts of similar marriage duration) who bear this strain. Row 3 of Table 4.8 fits in well with the above findings. The percentage of women currently pregnant is substantially higher for Tamil Nadu in the younger and therefore more briefly married age-group, but much lower for the older women.

Next we shall consider the closed birth interval proper, that is, the gap between one birth and the next. Row 2 of Table 4.8 indicates that there are few regional differences in mean inter-birth intervals and this variable is therefore not likely to be an important determinant of fertility differences in the two groups. We reach the same conclusion from the large national survey on inter-birth intervals conducted by the Registrar General of India (1988*b*). The mean closed interval was virtually identical in Tamil Nadu and Uttar Pradesh; the only difference was that, at about 43 months, it was substantially higher than in our study population. Similarly, the WFS (see McDonald 1984) found that there was very little difference in the mean length of inter-birth intervals among women marrying at different ages, at least for women aged 40–49 at the time of the survey. This was consistent with the small observed variations in the length of breast-feeding in the last closed interval according to the age at marriage.

But in the Indian case, similar intervals do not mean that there are no differences in the two primary determinants of birth intervals—lactation and contraceptive use—and one can see how a tilt in the balance between the two could lead to significant regional differentials in the gap between births. To begin with breast-feeding, row 4 of Table 4.8 finds a mean duration of breast-feeding for all children surviving until the date of the survey (a variable based on all live births would be hopelessly complicated by the multiple interactions between breast-feeding, amenor-rhoea, and child mortality) of 26 months for Uttar Pradesh and 20 months for Tamil Nadu. This is not a small difference and, using the observed relations in Bongaarts (1983), should lead to a difference of about three months in the duration of post-partum amenorrhoea. Of course, lactational infecundability is not a function of breast-feeding alone; the frequency and intensity of breast-feeding are also very important. But in the present case, regional differences in these latter variables are, if anything, in the direction of an even greater duration of infecundability for the Uttar Pradesh women than that predicted by equal frequency of suckling. For example, partial breast-feeding begins earlier in the Tamil households than in those from Uttar Pradesh: solids are introduced at about 10 months in the former and 13 months in the latter case, the difference being even greater for the older women.

How then do the Tamil Nadu women manage to achieve similar inter-birth intervals to their North Indian counterparts? The answer is contraception. The last three rows of Table 4.8 high-light regional differences in contraceptive use. Not only is the percentage of ever-users of contraception substantially higher in the South Indian women, the level of use of the more relevant modern non-terminal (that is, spacing) methods (the condom, IUD, and pill) is also much higher. State-level data (Ministry of Health and Family Welfare 1988) confirm this pattern. The regional difference in my study is the largest in the younger age-groups, which are the groups involved in active childbearing. For example, over three times as many women from Tamil Nadu as from Uttar Pradesh are current users of a modern method of contraception. Even more interestingly, as many as 18 per cent of the women who said that they wanted another child were found to be using a modern non-terminal method of contraception (implying that they were definitely thinking in terms of spacing), while for the Uttar Pradesh sample, this figure was 4 per cent. Add to this the finding that among such users the less effective condom is the most common method among the North Indian households, whereas for the Tamil women it is the much more effective IUD, and it is easy to see why the latter end up with as large birth intervals as the former. However, it needs to be noted that, for both groups, inter-birth intervals are substantially shorter than they are in the rural areas of the two regions of origin of our study population. Temporary birth-control is therefore a less than effective substitute for the decreased breast-feeding associated with our urban and more modern sample.

What does all this say about cultural influences on the pace of childbearing? Nothing in any direct sense, because there are no cultural differentials in the pace of childbearing. But once one looks at the determinants of this speed of childbearing, one can see the effect of kinship patterns and women's economic activities on the level of modernization expressed through shorter breast-feeding as well as through the greater use of modern temporary birth-control in the South Indian group. I discuss this issue more fully in the next section because the mechanisms involved are similar to those which lead to regional or cultural differentials in the termination of childbearing.

While this finding that changes in fertility are better explained by changes in the control of marital fertility rather than in birth intervals, is similar to that obtained by the Princeton European Fertility Project (see Knodel and van de Walle 1986), it must be mentioned that there does seem to be a growing body of literature which suggests that even sustained historical fertility declines may have had an element of deliberate control of the first as well as subsequent birth intervals (see, in particular, David and Sanderson 1987; Crafts 1989; Bean, Mineau, and Anderton 1990), at least in the USA and in England and Wales.

The Termination of Childbearing

Finally we come to regional differentials in the termination of childbearing. Table 4.9 sets out some indices of termination (rows 1 to 5) and some measures of the means of termination (rows 6 and 7) and the conclusion is inescapable: there are strong regional differentials in the woman's decision to cease childbearing. Even though inter-birth (that is, closed) intervals are similar, there are marked differences in the mean length of the open interval (for a similar state-level pattern, see Registrar General of India, 1988*b*), especially in the 30–49 year age-group, which is the age range during which a conscious decision to terminate childbearing is usually made. If we assume that an open interval of five years or more is a measure of the cessation of childbearing, row 2 of Table 4.9 confirms the regional differential. Alternatively, the mean number of births in the last five years (row 3) is also smaller for the Tamil women.

Is this earlier halt to childbearing among the Tamil women due to differences in natural fertility? It is in part, in one specific way. There are sharp regional differences in the proportion of women who cannot bear another child because of marriage disruption due to widowhood or separation (see Table 4.10). But these latter

Table 4.9. Regional differentials in the termination of childbearing

| | Uttar Pradesh (N=642) | | | | Tamil Nadu (N=578) | | | |
| | Age-group | | | | Age-group | | | |
	15–29	30–49	50+	All ages	15–29	30–49	50+	All ages
Mean length of open interval, in months	23	86	247	65	29	113	257	93
% women with no births in last 5 years	38	38	43	38	42	46	45	44
Mean number of births in last 5 years	1.9	0.8	0.1	1.3	1.7	0.5	0.0	1.1
% women who do not want another child	35	77	100	57	56	95	100	77
% women who say they cannot have another child	14	58	100	38	24	74	100	52
% women where either spouse is sterilized	7	35	17	21	21	53	9	33
% women practising terminal abstinence	0	0	0	0	0	1	2	1

Table 4.10. Regional differentials in exposure to pregnancy status

Age-group	% women who can bear another child[a]	% women who cannot bear another child because				
		Widowed or separated	Too old, or either spouse ill	Terminal abstinence	Other reasons	Either spouse sterilized
		Uttar Pradesh (N=642)				
15–29	85.6	1.6	2.6	0.0	3.5	6.7
30–49	42.2	3.9	14.4	0.0	5.9	33.7
50 +	0.0	34.8	52.2	0.0	0.0	13.0
All ages	61.7	3.4	10.0	0.0	5.1	19.8
		Tamil Nadu (N=578)				
15–29	75.7	2.5	0.7	0.0	0.7	20.5
30–49	26.3	14.2	7.1	1.3	2.1	49.0
50 +	0.0	64.3	33.9	1.8	0.0	0.0
All ages	48.0	13.3	6.6	0.7	1.2	30.3

[a] Including currently pregnant women.

differences are cultural rather than biological, since Tamil husbands do not have an unduly high mortality. The difference is
because (*a*) North Indian widows may face lower survival chances
than their southern counterparts (see Drèze 1990) (*b*) Tamil
couples do have a higher rate of separation and (*c*) on widowhood
or separation, the Tamil woman is more likely to continue to lead
her own life rather than return to the fold of her affinal kin in the
village of origin. All three patterns are a reflection of the greater
autonomy and potential for economic freedom of the South
Indian women, as well as their greater continued interaction with
the natal kin, characteristics which their cultural background
confers on them as discussed in earlier chapters.

But there also seem to be marked cultural differentials in
volitional fertility control. For one thing, there are very clear
regional differences in the proportion of women who say that they
do not want to have another child (row 4 of Table 4.9); there seems
to be a greater consciousness among the Tamil women about
stopping further pregnancies. This consciousness fits in well with
the larger proportions of Tamil women who feel that they cannot
have another child. Moreover, the regional differences in these
numbers are very large even for the youngest (15–29 year)
age-group, which is unlikely to be infertile for natural reasons
(except for primary sterility, of course, but we find no cultural
differences in the proportions of childless couples). Table 4.10 on
exposure status and row 6 of Table 4.9 suggest that terminal
contraception, that is, sterilization, is the largest contributor to
differences in the timing of the termination of childbearing. If we
add to this the regionally different figures on the percentages
of women using effective non-terminal birth-control (row 7 of
Table 4.8), the gap between women who desire no more births and
women who do something to achieve this desire gets relatively
narrowed for the South Indian sample.

The overall conclusion therefore is that volitional fertility
control is a major cause of cultural differences in marital fertility.
This is even more the case when one looks at the broader picture
of the two states as a whole, where the widowed or separated
North Indian woman with her curtailed exposure to pregnancy is
included as much in overall fertility estimates as is her South
Indian counterpart. Moreover, it is one specific kind of volitional
fertility control, the termination of childbearing, that is of greatest

importance. Although we agree with Hobcraft (1985) that a distinction between spacing and termination of births is not very realistic in most WFS countries, in the Indian case, where sterilization is the primary method of birth-control, we find that it does make sense to distinguish between the two, and that differentials are particularly marked in stopping behaviour.

4.3. Motivations

So much for the intermediate variables of fertility. A major conclusion in the last section was that fertility differences in our two cultural groups are the outcome of intentional fertility control rather than the result of differences in natural fertility. What accounts for these regional differences in intentional fertility control? External factors such as the presence of a strong family-planning programme in the home states of Uttar Pradesh and Tamil Nadu are certainly important, at least up to a point. But in our Delhi slum respondents have similar access to information and services related to family planning and in fact their similar socio-economic circumstances mean that, if one accepts the standard micro-economic literature on the subject, they often have similar needs to limit family size. And yet they behave differently.

Perhaps one should not so easily dismiss a structural explanation for these observed fertility differentials. After all most secondary sources suggest (and our own data confirm) significant fertility differentials by socio-economic variables such as household economic status, maternal education, and maternal occupation. And even if they do not offer a complete explanation of regional fertility differences, these factors do say a lot on the subject of fertility differentials, trends, and prospects within regional groups. However, before going any further one needs to add the caveat that since our sample is restricted to the urban poor, the range for the socio-economic variables is rather narrow. But in a sense this is also an advantage because it reinforces our point that cultural differences in demographic behaviour persist after controlling for non-region-specific socio-economic factors.

As in the chapters on child mortality, we use the potent example of maternal education to illustrate the role of socio-economic factors in fertility levels. The education–fertility link occupies paramount position in the demographic literature, and any attempt to single out a few specific studies would be futile in the present context: with varying degrees of refinement the broad finding remains that maternal education is associated with lower fertility.[5]

Table 4.11 agrees, even though we use a simple dichotomous variable of 'no education' and 'some education'. But more interesting than this straightforward relationship are two striking findings in Table 4.11

1. As in the maternal education–child mortality case discussed in the following chapter, the educational differential in fertility (and in its major proximate determinant, contraceptive use) is significantly greater for Uttar Pradesh than for Tamil Nadu. And, as in the education–mortality case, we advance two reasons for this regional pattern. First, the educated women from Uttar Pradesh represent a biased group distinguished by other innovative characteristics besides their exposure to a few years of schooling.

Table 4.11. Fertility indicators related to
maternal education

Fertility indicator	Maternal education	Uttar Pradesh (N=642)	Tamil Nadu (N=578)
Mean number of children ever born	None	4.1	3.6
	Some	2.2	3.0
	None/some	1.86	1.20
Total marital fertility rate	None	6.5	5.6
	Some	5.3	4.7
	None/some	1.23	1.19
% women who have ever used family planning	None	28	48
	Some	39	59
	None/some	0.71	0.81
% women who have ever used modern non-terminal contraception	None	8	19
	Some	28	28
	None/some	0.29	0.67

Secondly, the Tamil women as a whole represent a biased group distinguished by a relatively low fertility base to which education can contribute only up to a point. Moreover, education being relatively more universal among the Tamil women, the new norms associated with it have spread to the uneducated women as well.

2. Within each educational category, the current fertility of Tamil women is substantially lower (and contraceptive practice correspondingly higher) than that of our Uttar Pradesh respondents. This is in spite of the fact that among the women with some education, the North Indian women have higher levels of education than their Tamil counterparts. This suggests strongly that regional differences in the distribution of women according to education are not the main cause of observed differences in regional fertility.

We find the same thing when we look at other possible socio-economic determinants such as caste and maternal occupation: whatever the nature of the link, within each socio-economic category Tamil fertility is decidedly lower than that of Uttar Pradesh, therefore ruling out a prominent role for these variables in explaining overall regional differentials in fertility. Such a diminution of role is also suggested by the finding that these variables (except for education) often do not have similar effects in the two groups. For example, in the 30–49 year age-group, while working women from Uttar Pradesh have distinctly higher fertility than non-working women, for the Tamil Nadu women the reverse is true. As discussed elsewhere (see Basu and Sundar 1988), this is probably because of the nature of the occupation; but similar anomalies occur for other socio-economic indicators such as caste and income as well. And we are not alone in this. Even the World Fertility Survey (Singh and Casterline 1985), when it tried to put together the findings from different countries, found the socio-economic variables–fertility link to be hopelessly confused. The principle of anonymity did not seem to operate at all; each country needed to define its own unique relationship. This brings us back to regional or cultural factors which are important mediators in the relations between various indicators of socio-economic status and fertility behaviour.

To return to the persistence of fertility differences between regions even after controlling for socio-economic status, in this too

we are not alone. Cleland (1985) in an analysis of total marital
fertility rates according to father's occupation and rates of contraceptive use according to mother's education in twenty WFS
countries found that, in both cases, while there were important
socio-economic differences in these fertility indicators, the magni-
tudes of intra-country differences in such fertility indicators were
largely maintained within each socio-economic category. That is,
for example, if the national Total Marital Fertility Rate is lower in
Costa Rica than in Panama, the Total Marital Fertility Rate for
agricultural workers is also lower in Costa Rica than in Panama,
as is that for urban manual workers or urban white-collar workers.
Similarly, if current levels of contraceptive use are higher in
Colombia than in Paraguay, then they are also higher in the same
way for each category of maternal education. Which means that
observed differences in reproductive behaviour are not explained
by differences in the socio-economic composition of countries.

Other analyses of countries currently experiencing a demographic transition confirm this role of culture in fertility
behaviour. The general finding seems to be that sub-national
variations in fertility based on ethnic, religious, or linguistic
grounds persist strongly after controlling for possible confounding factors such as education and economic condition (see
for example, Alam and Cleland 1981; Soeradji and Hatmadji
1982; Gastardo-Conaco, Ramos-Jimenez, and Barniego 1986).
Historical data also support this hypothesis. The Princeton European Fertility Project (Coale and Watkins 1986) repeatedly
notes the importance of cultural and linguistic boundaries in
determining regional patterns of fertility change.[6]

All this suggests that differences in the micro-economic realities
of households can explain at best only a part of the regional
differential in fertility; and we borrow unabashedly and gratefully
from a paper by Cleland and Wilson (1987) which argues that
ideational rather than structural economic change is the main
force behind a fertility transition. In their words 'In our view, the
most striking feature of the onset of transition is its relationship to
broad cultural groupings. The spread of knowledge and ideas
seems to offer a better explanation for the observed pattern than
structural determinism.' Or, quoting Haines (1989) in the context
of the British fertility transition, 'People needed a change in their
basic outlook to consider substantial control of marital fertility as
a possible and worthwhile strategy.'

Two more lines of thought add weight to such an interpretation of fertility change over time or cross-sectional cultural differences in fertility. The first is the strength of the inverse education–fertility relationship, which remains little affected by controls for the socio-economic circumstances of the household including (especially) maternal employment. Moreover, the effect emerges even for women with a few years of schooling, suggesting that education does not lead to lower fertility because of changes in the costs and benefits of children but because of changes in ideas. The role of diffusion processes for new ideas (Cleland (1985) calls this 'social imitation') is also suggested by our survey finding that socio-economic differentials in fertility are smaller in our Tamil than in our Uttar Pradesh sample, which is further behind in the demographic transition. But socio-economic differentials in the structural factors affecting the demand for children remain and yet demographic behaviour in the different socio-economic groups tends to converge, implying that it is more the adoption of innovative ideas that is responsible. The experience of other areas is similar: the speed with which fertility decline seems to spread to all sections of a culturally homogeneous population, in both historical and currently developing countries, tends to be out of all proportion to the possible speed of changes in the micro-economic realities of households.

So much for establishing the importance of culture in explaining regional fertility differences. But culture is an amorphous concept and what this chapter has tried to do is to find some connections between specific aspects of the culture in the North–South context and the proximate determinants of fertility. The stress was on regional differentials in marriage and kinship patterns and in the employment of women. In turn, these cultural factors are associated with regional differences in the position of women. Note that a definition of the 'position of women' here does not attempt any normative rankings; it only describes certain characteristics relevant to fertility behaviour. For example it is quite plausible that when women in the higher classes in North India withdraw from the labour-force with increased household income, their incentive to control their fertility falls but their social status rises.

While our findings on cultural differences in the position of women in ways relevant for demographic behaviour have been discussed in earlier chapters, it would be worthwhile to restate here the three related ways in which our Tamil Nadu women differ from our Uttar Pradesh respondents:

(*a*) greater exposure to the outside world;
(*b*) greater interaction with the outside world; and
(*c*) greater autonomy in decision-making.

According to our hypothesis, these differences in female position lead to regional differences in fertility of course, but, much more interestingly, they are reflected in regional differences in those proximate determinants of fertility most closely related to female attitudes and knowledge as opposed to purely household or community characteristics. Table 4.12 summarizes these results well and is only worth paraphrasing on a few specific points.

The first of these is the assumption that a non-numeric response to a numerical question says something about female status. We believe it does. Not only is a minimum level of numeracy essential for parity-specific birth-control to be possible (that is, numeracy is essential for fertility to come, to quote Coale 1973, 'within the calculus of conscious choice'), functional numeracy also indirectly affects the woman's responses to everyday life, especially those situations involving the making of decisions. The spread of such numeracy is a recent phenomenon and it is therefore not surprising that it is much more common in the younger than in the older women for both groups. What is much more interesting is the finding that even the oldest Tamil women were more likely to give a numerical response to questions on ideal family size than were the youngest age-groups from Uttar Pradesh.

As for actual birth-control practice, it has already been mentioned that sterilization levels are higher in the Tamil households. However, sterilization is the main method offered by the official family-planning programme and its acceptance is related to several other factors besides the role of women (the persuasive powers of the government, for example). But the use of modern non-terminal contraception is much more connected with individual knowledge and decision-making and here once again (see row 4 of Table 4.12) the South Indian women score well above their North Indian counterparts, especially in the 15–29 year age-group.

Not only is sterilization the main method pushed by the family-planning programme but it is almost exclusively female

Table 4.12. Fertility indicators related to the position of women

| | Uttar Pradesh (N=642) | | | | Tamil Nadu (N=578) | | |
| | Age-group | | | | Age-group | | |
	15–29	30–49	50+	All ages	15–29	30–49	50+	All ages
Mean desired family size	3.46	3.54	3.69	3.50	2.66	2.98	3.48	2.86
% women giving a non-numeric response to question on ideal family size	20	24	44	23	3	8	18	6
% women who think a small family has no advantages	20	18	30	19	5	11	30	10
% women who have ever used modern non-terminal birth-control	15	10	0	12	33	14	2	22
% women whose husbands are sterilized	2	14	4	8	2	23	4	11
% never-users who think they will use birth-control in the future	17	13	0	15	58	17	0	36

sterilization which is emphasized (see Basu 1985). It therefore comes as no great surprise (given the trend of our findings so far) that in the peak sterilization age-group of 30–49, male sterilization levels are substantially higher among the Tamilian households. While this is certainly partly due to the greater amenability of the Tamil male (and the greater shame attached to a male sterilization in the North Indian machismo culture), it is also a reflection of the greater power that Tamil wives wield within the household. Their frequent economic indispensability is one factor, but equally important is their overall greater equality in decision-making on household matters, so that it is less naturally assumed that the entire responsibility for birth-control rests with them.

The overall impression from Table 4.12 is that the women from Tamil Nadu have much clearer (and lower) fertility goals than the women from Uttar Pradesh and their actions to meet these goals are also more deliberate and effective. There are sub-group variations in both these variables of course, but these are smaller than the variations between the two regional groups. It is not clear if these lower fertility desires of the South Indians can be attributed solely to either structural factors or to the diffusion of modern ideas. While we have gone to some lengths in the last several paragraphs to suggest that structural factors are not important, perhaps it should be clarified that by structural factors we mean simply the economic position of the household and the extra-domestic options that confront the household. For, even when these are similar for both regional groups, fertility differences exist. But it is of course true at the same time that the demand for children is also influenced by structural factors, in that the extent to which women affect or respond to (both in effect as well as only potentially) these household and environmental characteristics influences the overall need for children. But the point is that these aspects of women's position are in turn affected more by their cultural background than by their immediate circumstances.

At this point it would be useful to try and tease out a more tangible connection between women's status and fertility desires. I think the crucial cultural variable is the cultural difference in the demand for sons. Indeed, this whole question of 'son preference' in India deserves a special section because of the ways in which it is linked not only to fertility but, as importantly, to the intra-household sex differential in welfare that exists in South Asia as a whole and the northern part of this region in particular. We therefore briefly turn to this subject now.

4.4. Son Preference and Regional Differences in Son Preference

The circumstances which support a higher demand for sons in India are essentially the same as those which support a higher demand for children in high fertility areas in general, only stronger. Therefore, if value-of-children data suggest that there is an economic case to be made for having relatively more children, in the South Asian context this is almost always a case for having relatively more sons. Similarly, if child replacement and insurance effects lead to a higher demand for children in high mortality situations, the demand for additional children is likely to be even greater when the dead child is male or where the perceived mortality of sons is high.

How do we know that there is a strong relative preference for sons in India? From several kinds of qualitative as well as quantitative evidence. To begin with, there is the mass of anecdotal or descriptive material both in the creative arts as well as in ethnographic or anthropological accounts of life in this region which brings out the strong desire in women as well as households as a whole for one or more sons. To give a trivial but nevertheless potent example, every observer or resident of the Indian scene has personal knowledge of at least a handful of homes where childbearing has continued mercilessly until a son has been born, even when this means a string of five, six, or even seven and more daughters first. On the other hand, we would be hard put to identify even one home which has as many sons and a youngest daughter whose late arrival has been the main reason for repeated pregnancies and with whose birth childbearing comes to an end.

Coming to more quantitative evidence, first there is the indirect kind suggested by the marked sex differentials in mortality and other aspects of child welfare in much of the Indian sub-continent. A sex ratio of child mortality adverse to girls has been commented on for some decades now (see, for example,

Visaria, 1967) and there is no longer much interest in this general question in either the census or a survey; the focus of attention is now on the finer details of this sex difference in mortality and the factors responsible for it. But whatever these details and these factors, the essential conclusion is that, given the premise that girls are biologically at least as hardy as, if not hardier than, boys, their higher death-rates suggest a greater preoccupation with the existence and survival of boys. The increasing popularity of the amniocentesis procedure to detect and subsequently abort the female foetus is just one more expression of this fact that a large proportion of deliberate pregnancies in the country are entered into because of the desire for a first or additional son.

We also have more direct quantitative evidence of this Indian pattern of sex preference. In survey after survey of the KAP (knowledge, attitudes, and practices) type, answers to questions about ideal family size and the ideal sex composition of families lead to the same conclusion—that couples would be much more likely to restrict fertility if they achieved a minimum of one or two living sons, ideally two or three. For example, the Operation Research Group's second all-India survey of family-planning practices (Khan and Prasad 1983) found that as many as 57 per cent of respondents felt that the best sex composition of children was one which had two or more sons and varying numbers of daughters (never exceeding the number of sons). As expected, this figure hides a significant urban–rural differential, with 60 per cent of rural respondents favouring such a sex composition as opposed to a lower (but still remarkably high) 47 per cent in the urban areas.

But then people do not necessarily practise what they preach, especially in the area of family planning, where survey respondents have been quick to learn ideal survey responses and where few KAP surveys have been unable to demonstrate a strong positive commitment to family planning and the small family norm even when actual levels of contraceptive use leave much to be desired. But even when we look at actual fertility-control behaviour, the data are surprisingly consistent with stated sex preferences. Unfortunately Ministry of Health and Family Welfare statistics do not provide the sex composition of children of contraceptive acceptors, but it is revealing that the number of living children of sterilization acceptors is consistently closer to three than to the officially promoted two (one would be willing to bet that this achieved family size of three living children largely consists of at least two sons). However, the Operations Research Group survey mentioned above does provide such information. The proportion of couples who have accepted a sterilization jumps sharply as the number of living sons rises from zero to one and even more sharply when it goes up to two. Even more interesting is the relation between the number of living sons and the use of any form of contraception (not just sterilization). Here too the fall in the number of never-users is very sharp as one goes from zero to one and one to two surviving sons. This suggests that the hurry to bear sons does not even allow the use of temporary or spacing methods between pregnancies.

We come next to the reasons for such a sex preference and to the related question of whether it is more marked in the northern part of the country: is there a regional differential in sex preference which is at least partly responsible for the regional differential in the overall demand for children? We already have much evidence of a North–South difference in the sex ratio in childhood mortality; as discussed in the last chapter, this is much more strongly against girls in the northern part of the country. More directly, in the present study the mean number of sons considered ideal was 2.16 in the Uttar Pradesh sample and 1.69 in the Tamil sample. And it was this difference which explained the difference in ideal family size between the two groups: the desire for daughters was similar (at about 1.3) in the two groups. Secondary data confirm this pattern. For instance, Khan and Prasad's all-India survey (1983) found that about 70 per cent of respondents in the northern region of the country felt that the ideal family should have at least two sons, while the corresponding figure for the southern zone was 40 per cent. Bhatia (1978) reported similar regional differences in son preference from his state-level data on ideal family size. Similarly, in large-scale surveys in the North Indian states of Bihar and Rajasthan, Kanitkar and Murthy (1983) found that the number of surviving sons had the largest influence on the ever-use of contraceptive methods in both states, larger even than the effect of that other potent variable, maternal education. And Khan and Gupta (1987) reported that as many as 57 per cent of the respondents in their

Uttar Pradesh study were prepared to have three or more daughters just to get a second (not first) son, compared to a figure of 20 per cent for the country as a whole.

The preference for sons is greater in the northern states for the same reasons that the demand for children is greater in this area, with the variable of women's socio-economic dependence on men being even more important than it is for determining overall demand for children because, in a situation where women have less of an independent existence, additional daughters are no additional source of security to the woman or to her household. To state briefly the conditions under which the demand for sons would be greater: first, son preference is likely to be strong for economic reasons where the labour-market is more segmented by sex. In that case, sons may be needed as a source of economic gain as well as support against economic loss. For example, sons may be needed to prevent the loss of income caused by inadequate utilization of land because many agricultural activities are barred to women, as well as to exploit successfully the potential gains from migration in a situation where rural–urban migration is primarily young-male selective. Such labour-market segmentation increases the economic value of sons to the household as a whole. In addition, one extreme form of sex segmentation of the labour-market—when access to productive employment is barred to women not just in certain specific activities, but in virtually all activities, making women economically dependent on men— independently increases the woman's demand for sons as support in the possible absence of economic support from the husband for reasons such as death, desertion, or debility (see Cain 1982). While sex segmentation of the labour-market exists in most parts of traditional South Asia, the virtual exclusion of women from the labour-force as a whole is confined to very specific regions, in particular those occupying the north and north-western part of India. It is therefore little wonder that the sex preference variable is also the strongest in this region.

Certain other cultural traditions also make sons more necessary or valuable. For example, most traditional South Asian cultures stress the role of the son in looking after his parents. But in some cultures (again more prominent in northern India), this re-sponsibility of the sons is strengthened by the greater severance of ties with a married daughter. Such relatively greater severance in

North India is facilitated by the practice of village and kin exogamy in marriage (see Dyson and Moore 1983); by the very clear emotional and functional distinction between the daughter and the daughter-in-law (see Mandelbaum 1988*b*; Karve 1965); by the tradition which sees the parents of the bride as the givers and those of the groom as the takers; and by the status of the woman in her household being determined by the level of her allegiance to her affinal kin. Such cultural differences in the level of post-marital contact between a woman and her parents naturally lead to differences in the value attached to sons as the ultimate source of economic and social security.

Contrary to most lay opinion on the subject, there are few religious reasons to explain the strong preference for sons in India. The majority, or, Hindu religion provides remarkably many fairly easy solutions to the religious problems that sonlessness can present. For example, even the funeral rites for which the scriptures require a son can, in the absence of such an available son, be alternatively performed by one from a long list of substitute relations arranged in some descending order of preference by the keepers of the religion.

How does son preference affect final fertility? While most traditional analyses have tended to conclude that the two are positively related, using data from China, where there is a very strong preference for at least one son, Arnold and Zhaoxieng (1986) made some more direct calculations to conclude that such son preference has only a small effect on contraceptive use as the vast majority of couples have at least one son in their childbearing years by sheer chance (only about one in eight couples who have children have only daughters). In a later paper, Arnold (1987) applied this method to estimate the effects of son preference to fertility to several other countries and reached the same conclusion that the removal of son preference can be expected to have only very modest effects on fertility. While his calculations seem watertight, I have several problems with his interpretations.

To begin with, actual contraceptive behaviour is affected by several other factors besides son preference. For instance, the Chinese experience is unique in that overall contraceptive use rates are so high (for whatever reason), being for example around 65 per cent even for women with only one child, that there is less scope for son preference to assert itself (there is an implicit

acknowledgement of this in the author's finding that son preference seemed to have had a significantly greater effect on fertility
in the past). In contrast, the other detailed example in the paper
refers to the Menoufia Governorate in Egypt, where even couples
who presumably have as many sons as they would like never
seem to reach contraceptive use rates of more than about 30 per
cent. The author is aware of this and tries to repeat the analysis
by aggregating countries according to overall levels of contraceptive use, and reaches essentially similar results. But then, such
aggregation leads to a selection bias in that the countries with the
greatest son preference tend to fall in the group with the lowest
rates of contraceptive use.

Ideally we need to look at a situation in which son preference
is held constant but the other constraints on contraceptive use are
removed. To take an extreme example, consider a situation in
which one group of women desires at least one son and the other
at least two, and that both groups stop further childbearing
completely once these minima are achieved. We could call these
two groups the South Indians and the North Indians for convenience and without too great a departure from reality. Using
the sex composition distributions at different parities in Arnold's
Egypt example, such behaviour implies that:

(*a*) among women with one child, no North Indians will terminate further childbearing, while 51 per cent of the South
Indians will;

(*b*) among women with two children, 28 per cent of the North
Indians and 80 per cent of the South Indians will cease further
childbearing;

(*c*) among women with three children, 58 per cent of the North
Indians and 91 per cent of the South Indians will stop
reproduction.

These differences are substantial by any reckoning and fertility
differences become even greater when we consider that for a given
base level of women, not only are rates of birth-control use higher
among the South Indians for equivalent parity, the absolute
numbers of the South Indian women are also much smaller at each
parity above one.

Arnold's main result seems to be biased by the fact that while he
discusses the situation of changed sex preferences with existing
levels of contraceptive use, he is not able to consider the parallel

situation of unchanged (or more clearly specified) sex preferences but more effective contraceptive use. Such a comment has been made in Cleland, Verrall, and Vaessen (1983) based on World Fertility Survey data which found a high level of son preference in the South Asian region and a corresponding positive fertility response. The authors speculate that as birth-control becomes more common in this region, the effect of son preference on fertility will almost certainly increase.

There is another problem with such analyses. This is the use of the number of living children as a proxy for fertility. It is justified if one is concerned with the effect of son preference on aggregate population growth rates, but less so when one is talking about the woman herself and her fertility as defined by the number of live births and not the number of living children. In such a case, when one considers, say, the woman with three living children, one is probably referring to a number of live births which is greater than three, the difference between the two being a function of the mortality level of young boys.

Therefore, in the Indian kind of situation, where anticipated child loss is high and the general preference is for at least two sons, as voluntary fertility control becomes more widespread, overall fertility will have to be considerably higher to satisfy prevailing sex preferences than it would have been in the absence of such preferences. The chances of getting two sons in any given number of pregnancies are smaller than those of getting only one son; and the chances of having two sons that survive childhood are even smaller for any given number of pregnancies. For example, May and Heer (1968) estimated in the 1960s that for an Indian couple to have a 98 per cent probability of raising one son to adulthood, they had to have over six births. And if the preference is for two or more sons, as our review of the available literature has shown, one can see why the official family-planning programme has not got very far in its policy of promoting a two-child norm. As Bose (1988) stressed, the official perception of this norm means one son and one daughter, or two sons and no daughter, or no son and two daughters; whereas the people, who also agree with the view that a small family is a happy family, take a small family to mean two sons and one daughter or two sons and no daughter, and 'since one cannot order only two sons, family building continues until two sons arrive and it also continues until two sons survive'.

Gulati's (1987) study confirms the existence of such a family-building strategy. His data are from Delhi and therefore re-presentative of the northern part of the country. Keeping the value of other influences on the desire for additional children fixed at their mean values in the study sample, he found that the probability of wanting another child was 0.67 for couples with one son and one daughter, 0.61 for couples with one son and two daughters, but only 0.47 for couples with two sons and one daughter. Even in families with four living children, the pro-bability was 0.55 if the couple had one son and three daughters, but only 0.28 if it had three sons and one daughter.

The discussion so far about the value of sons should not be interpreted to mean that there is no demand for daughters. The usual situation is for couples to want one daughter even for economic reasons. It is the daughter who is useful for performing specific chores, especially within the home and especially where there is no cultural or other compulsion to keep her in school. There is also a ritual merit in having a daughter to give away in marriage. The desire for a daughter is well brought out in the Khan and Prasad (1983) survey which found that in three-child families, only 11 per cent of couples with two sons and one daughter wanted another child, whereas 23 per cent of those with three sons and no daughter wanted an additional birth.

However, these positive aspects of daughters fall sharply with additional daughters and negative factors become paramount, as is seen, for example, in Das Gupta's (1987) finding in Punjab that the sex differential in child mortality is much higher for second and subsequent daughters. Moreover, for all daughters including the first, the anticipated marriage costs are an important factor influencing the demand for them. However, even here there are important regional differences, which is why Khan and Prasad (1983) reported that in the South the proportion of families that thought that an ideal family would have as many daughters as sons was 65 per cent but only 37 per cent in the northern region of the country. Unfortunately, we do not have data in this study on people's reactions to daughterless families, but available evidence suggests that these would be fairly negative in any part of the country.

We can do no better than to end this section with a quote from the epic of Gilgamesh, which is believed to be the oldest recorded literary work in any language. Set in ancient Mesopotamia, the central character's quest for immortality is answered thus by his friend from the underworld, who makes reference to the situation of man upon death:

'Have you seen the man who has no son?'
  'I have seen him.
He ...'   (*indecipherable in the original tablets*)
'The one with one son: have you seen him?'
  'I have seen him.
He lies under the wall, weeping bitterly.'
'The one with two sons: have you seen him?'
  'I have.
He lives in a brick house and eats bread.'
                              (Gardner and Maier, 1985)

The descriptions get progressively more cheerful as the friend describes the dead with more and more sons, until

'The one with six sons: have you seen him?'
  'I have.
Like the man who guides the plough, he feels pride.'
'The one with seven sons; have you seen him?'
  'I have.
Like a man close to the gods, he ...'
                    (*indecipherable in the original tablets*)

It appears that the Asian idea of dependence on children in general and sons in particular is neither new nor derived solely from a concern with immediate material goals.

4.5. The Men

If this chapter has so far made very little explicit reference to the other side of the reproductive partnership, the husband, the intention was not to deny a crucial role to men in family-building strategies and decisions. The attempt was the more modest one of illustrating that women's status has an important and independent bearing on these issues. Men's wishes play a complementary role, one which can become all-engulfing when the woman's authority declines. But it may be rewarding to consider this subject somewhat less cursorily at this point. Two separate but interrelated questions need to be addressed in this consideration of the relative roles of husbands and wives—

the extent to which men's and women's fertility goals differ,[7] and the extent to which actual behaviour is dictated by the preferences of one spouse over the other. In the current framework, the focus would be on how both these factors are affected by the status of women. The following discussion will perforce be brief and to a large extent speculative; hard statistics are difficult to come by.

On the empirical evidence on gender differentials in reproductive goals, Mason and Taj (1987) concluded from an extensive review of the literature that there are no clear patterns, although accepted theories of fertility motivations might lead us to deduce that there are clear differences in the need for children between husbands and wives. The only trouble is that different interpretations of theories give us as many reasons to expect differentials in one direction as in the other. In other words, as yet our theories do not seem to have much predictive value in the area of gender differences in family-size desires. The best strategy seems instead to be to determine gender differences empirically and then try to explain them. While there has been much implicit discussion in the literature on the reasons to expect men and women to have differing fertility goals, there has been less of an attempt to explain common goals in a traditional setting. It is therefore worth wondering why the empirical search by Taj and Mason found that gender differences in fertility goals were non-existent or small. One can think of several reasons for this (assuming of course that the findings are real and not a reflection of the quality or the marginal interest in the subject of the studies reviewed).

The most obvious interpretation is that husbands and wives do independently have similar fertility goals, because their motivations and background circumstances are similar. But if we realistically assume that this is not always the case, what could account for the observed commonality of family-size desires in the literature? First, as the authors of the review also discuss, it may be that most of the available literature refers to populations which are already undergoing a fertility transition, and it is in pre-transition societies that one would expect to find the greatest gender differentials. Secondly, since the review measured net differences between average family-size goals of husbands and wives, as opposed to the proportion of individual couples in which husbands and wives had differing goals, there may have been some tendency for sub-groups with a difference in one direction to be balanced out by those which differed in the other. If that is the case, it is not clear how important fertility goal differences are in aggregate reproductive behaviour. Thirdly, stated family-size ideals may be a reflection of behaviour rather than ante-dating and/or determining behaviour. But, of course, this does not apply to younger cohorts, for their family-size ideals would then be unacceptably low in several cases. But this is not an impossible argument for older couples, the literature on the 'wantedness of the last child' notwithstanding. Fourthly, family-size goals may be similar between spouses because both spouses have accepted and are stating the goals of the more powerful spouse. This kind of dominance is impossible to detect by the ordinary survey method and is understandably inferred from other kinds of evidence and theories about intra-household relationships. Finally, and this is a more generous variant of the fourth interpretation above, one may have a case of *folie à deux*. This translates literally as 'double madness' or the presence of the same or similar delusional ideas in two persons closely associated with each other. In the present context, it refers to a convergence of fertility goals between husband and wife, as the two influence and are influenced by each other, not necessarily through pressure but through persuasion and through constant exposure to each other's views and beliefs.

To return to the central theme of this book, in the context of the current section, the main conclusion would be that women's reproductive goals are an important predictor of men's goals and household reproductive behaviour because, for any one or more of the reasons detailed above, spousal differences in reproductive goals are likely to be small. In the present study, the mean family sizes desired by husbands and wives were virtually identical. But since the data concerning husbands' desires were obtained from the wives in the survey, it is always possible that we were not getting the complete truth. Moreover, even when they are similar but independently derived, both men's and women's fertility preferences are likely to be shaped by the position of women as defined in the present context. For example, in a situation of sex segmentation of the labour-market, or one of a severance of ties with married daughters, both men and women should have an increased demand for sons (and, by extension, for children) than in situations where these factors do not operate. Incidentally, this same kind of argument can be invoked to include other potentially important decision-makers in the family, such as the mother-in-law. And once goals are similar, the second question that was posed at the beginning of this section, concerning whose preferences determine behaviour, becomes somewhat irrelevant.

One must admit a feeling of dissatisfaction with this section; there is so much to know and so little to go on. One can only hope that this subject becomes a more important part of the research on intra-household relationships in the future.

4.6. Discussion

We are now able to expand the model of the status of women and demographic behaviour giving fertility as the component of demographic behaviour, as shown in Fig. 4.1

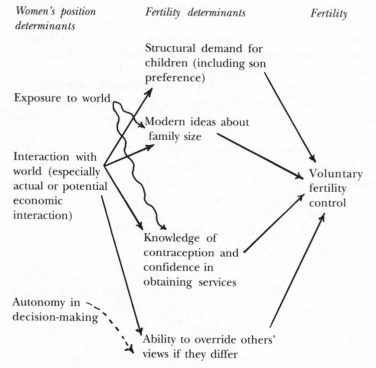

| *Women's position determinants* | *Fertility determinants* | *Fertility* |

Structural demand for children (including son preference)

Exposure to world

Modern ideas about family size

Interaction with world (especially actual or potential economic interaction)

Voluntary fertility control

Knowledge of contraception and confidence in obtaining services

Autonomy in decision-making

Ability to override others' views if they differ

FIG. 4.1. A model of the status of women and its influence on fertility

Note that the model in this form refers to the intermediate

variables which affect volitional fertility control, and not to those proximate determinants which influence 'natural' fertility. This is because of the finding in Section 4.2 that regional differentials in achieved fertility are a function of regional differentials in the termination of childbearing, with regional differences in the determinants of natural fertility tending to cancel one another out. We could, of course, include in the above model the effects of the position of women on these other potential proximate determinants of fertility, such as the age at marriage and birth-spacing behaviour, but as yet these seem to be only indirectly connected to final fertility levels through their influence on parity-specific birth-control, rather than having a direct effect on differences in non-parity specific fertility. Even the greater amount of contraceptive use between births by the South Indian women seems to be doing little other than compensating for the longer breast-feeding durations among the North Indians, with closed birth intervals being very similar in the two groups.

Besides the direct effect of the postulated components of women's position, there is the possible indirect effect of each component via its interaction with one or more of the other components. For example, while we cannot see why autonomy in decision-making should lead to a smaller structural demand for children, one can imagine a pathway of influence that goes something like this:

autonomy $\longrightarrow$ economic interaction with the outside world $\longrightarrow$ need for children as security.

Indeed, the bulk of the effect of female autonomy on the determinants of voluntary fertility control probably occurs through its effect on the two other components of women's position. In this sense it is much more powerful than our simple model suggests. At the same time, it should be stressed that while female autonomy often leads to greater exposure and/or interaction, it is not a necessary condition for them; they can exist even in the absence of women's control over their lives. For instance, other household members can have important altruistic or vested interests in sending girls to school or women to work, both factors contributing to their exposure to and interaction with the world outside the home. For the sake of simplicity, such indirect effects have not been spelt out in the formal model.

NOTES

1. Incidentally, larger-scale data sources such as the census support exactly this pattern of fertility differential between the states of Uttar Pradesh and Tamil Nadu.

2. There does not seem to be any indication from secondary sources that there are significant differences in the age at menarche between the two study groups. The primary data-set does not have information on this question.

3. As Coale (1991) has demonstrated, historically there has been a strong positive connection between the age at marriage and the use of birth-control to limit fertility. This is not so much because later marriage promotes birth-control as because 'the customs governing marriage and the formation of households affect both the age at marriage and the autonomy of young people, especially women'.

4. The problem is analogous to the apparent contradiction which exists between studies which show a positive relation at the aggregate level between hospital deliveries and child survival (for example, Jain 1985) and several micro-level analyses which are bewildered by a negative relation. The latter occurs usually because the data refer to areas where hospital deliveries are relatively rare and hospital births therefore include an unnaturally large proportion of high-risk or emergency cases.

5. However, there are some situations in which the association does not occur and situations in which it may be in the opposite direction. The latter is likely to happen at very low levels of development where the primary effect of education is the relaxation of traditional restraints of childbearing, and at high levels of development where higher education may increase incomes enough to make children more affordable. On all these points, see, among others, Graaf 1979; Cochrane 1979; Rodriguez and Cleland 1980; Nag 1980; United Nations Population Division 1983; Singh and Casterline 1985).

6. In all fairness one must note that the literature does also contain committed proponents of an 'adaptation' as opposed to an 'innovation/diffusion' explanation of traditional fertility transitions. See, in particular, Carlsson (1966) on the Swedish fertility transition and, more recently, Bean, Mineau, and Anderton (1990) on the Mormon demographic transition in the USA.

7. Note that we are talking about husband–wife differentials in family size desires, not about husband–wife differentials in the accurate reporting of behaviour. The latter has been considered in the literature (see, for example, Yaukey, Roberts, and Griffiths 1965).

5

Infant and Child Mortality

IT is already known from several sources of secondary information that there can be wide regional variations in levels of infant and child mortality. For example, in India the Registrar General of India's (1981a) survey of infant and child mortality found that for the 1978 birth cohort, infant mortality in rural Uttar Pradesh (172 per thousand live births) was 1.43 times higher than in rural Tamil Nadu and in the urban areas it (at 110 per thousand live births) was as much as 1.75 times higher than in urban Tamil Nadu. But then, Uttar Pradesh and Tamil Nadu are differentiated by much more than cultural context and the status of women. For example, they vary greatly in the level and kind of health facilities accessible to the general population (Department of Health and Family Welfare 1985) and at least somewhat in the unkindness of the physical environment. So it is difficult to know how far the above mortality differences are a reflection of differences in household-level attitudes and behaviour.

The present study allows some ways out of this impasse. By selecting respondent households of different cultural background but similar socio-economic circumstances and living in an identical physical environment, we are able to control to a large extent for the effect of extra-household variables and identify some of the ways in which the position of women affects the survival chances of children. Once more, a mix of quantitative and qualitative methods is used to understand the relationships involved.

While we do not want to anticipate the findings, which are summarised in Section 5.4, it is worth mentioning briefly (especially for those who would balk at the length of this chapter) that our evidence does indeed suggest several ways in which women's roles within and outside the home affect their ability to care for their children. Two more findings which are probably generalizable to other population groups stand out. First, that child health is an important priority in any cultural context and

Table 5.1. Regional differentials in childhood mortality[a]

	Uttar Pradesh	Tamil Nadu
q(2)	0.1979	0.1007
q(3)	0.1987	0.1983
q(5)	0.2429	0.2274
Average mortality level	12.59	15.01
Graduated q(2)[b]	0.1916	0.1538
Graduated q(3)[b]	0.2144	0.1701
Graduated q(5)[b]	0.2333	0.1836

[a] Using the South family of model life-tables and Trussell's equation

[b] Graduated q(x) values are the q(x) values in the South model life-table system corresponding to the average mortality level.

is reflected in the ease with which the modern health-care habit (except in very specific ways as brought out in the next chapter) is acquired for dealing with childhood illnesses once suitable health services become available. Secondly, a less encouraging but important finding is the potential negative impact of women's economic activity on child survival: poor working women, in spite of the other advantages of their work, seem to do worse on the child mortality front. However, we attempt to find intervention points to affect this unfortunate relationship in the intermediate mechanisms involved in the relationship, rather than unfairly condemning female employment as a source of child neglect.

5.1. Regional Differentials

In spite of the controls for socio-economic factors and the external environment, our data find the same regional pattern of child mortality as observed in the two states of origin. Table 5.1 presents indirect estimates of child mortality derived from data on children ever born and proportions dead and using Trussell's South model coefficients as described in the United Nations *Manual X* (1983). The graduated q(5) values suggest that the Uttar Pradesh child has a much greater probability of dying in early childhood than a Tamil child. Indeed, the contrast is probably sharper than it appears because of possible significant under-enumeration of dead daughters in the Uttar Pradesh sample, as discussed in the next chapter.

In spite of this region-selective under-reporting, Table 5.2 on direct measures of infant and child mortality continues to find the Uttar Pradesh child at a relatively greater disadvantage: we have 111 children from Uttar Pradesh dying for every 100 Tamil children who die. We explore the age-specific mortality, cohort mortality, and regional differentials evident in Table 5.2 in Section 5.4 of this chapter. Here, we first turn to the possible proximate determinants through which these regional mortality differentials emerge.

5.2. Mechanisms

Analogous to the literature on fertility determinants, recent research on child mortality has tried to understand variations in infant and child mortality in terms of differences in a group of 'proximate determinants'. The framework for doing this was first proposed formally by Mosley and Chen (1984) and Mosley (1985), who hypothesized that all socio-economic and cultural factors which influence child mortality do so through their effect on a set of intermediate variables which in turn directly influence the risk of morbidity and mortality. These proximate determinants were grouped by them into five categories: demographic factors, environmental contamination, nutrient deficiency, injury, and personal illness control. The relationship between child mortality and these proximate determinants is assumed to be fixed, basically on the premise that it is a biological or endogenous one. Instead, this chapter finds that the relation between child mortality and these proximate determinants is nowhere near as fixed as that between fertility and its proximate determinants, even when one looks at the so-called bio-demographic proximate determinants. That is, not only do socio-economic and socio-cultural factors affect child mortality by way of their effect on the proximate determinants, the proximate determinant–child mortality relationship itself is also mediated by socio-economic and socio-cultural factors.

The other major problem, of course, is that so many of the

Table 5.2. Regional differentials in childhood mortality: direct estimates

Mother's region of origin, and years since child's birth	% children dead	% children dying within[a]						age at death not stated
		1 week	1 month	1–11 months	1–4 years	1 year	5 years	
Uttar Pradesh (N=2482)								
0	7.5							
1–4	14.1	4.0	5.9	3.4		9.3		2.2
5–9	23.7	5.9	7.9	7.9	5.2	15.7	20.9	2.6
10–14	26.3	6.0	8.3	6.8	7.4	15.1	22.5	2.1
15+	38.5	8.1	11.3	9.8	11.2	21.1	32.3	3.8
Time of birth not stated	95.8	0.0	16.7	16.7	33.3	0.0	33.3	62.5
All ages	26.2	6.1	8.6	7.4	8.0	25.7	25.7	3.3
Tamil Nadu (N=2007)								
0	3.8							
1–4	13.9	4.3	4.0	4.8		10.2		0.8
5–9	21.2	4.2	5.7	7.3	5.7	13.0	18.9	1.9
10–14	25.1	3.4	4.3	8.3	10.3	12.6	22.9	0.9
15+	29.7	7.2	9.2	5.7	8.1	14.9	23.0	2.3
Time of birth not stated	100.0	0.0	0.0	0.0	0.0	0.0	0.0	100.0
All ages	23.6	5.3	6.8	6.3	7.9	21.7	21.7	2.0

[a] Each of columns 4 to 9 includes only those live births which occurred before the relevant age at death interval and could therefore have theoretically been exposed to death during that age interval.

proximate determinants are themselves heavily correlated, so that one would need very complicated regressions to prevent a certain amount of overestimation of effects. Nevertheless, this chapter is designed on the premise that there is also much to be learned from relatively simple analysis of the data. Firstly, because complicated and competent analyses of large data sets, on which one can peg the results of micro-studies such as the present one, already exist (see, in particular, Rutstein (1983); Hobcraft, McDonald, and Rutstein 1985). Secondly, even when a variable may be less directly connected to child survival than a simple relationship indicates, it is an important way of identifying a high-risk group, the underlying policy goal being an attempt to change the general conditions for this group quite apart from influencing merely the index variable. Thirdly, small-scale studies allow one to identify qualitatively the possible reasons for an observed relationship between child mortality and a seemingly proximate determinant.

It is in such a spirit that the following pages consider each of the intermediate variable categories of Mosley and Chen (1984) in turn and try to gauge their relative importance in explaining regional differences in infant and child mortality. It may be added that by looking only at the poor, the present study reduces substantially the confounding effects of socio-economic variables as determinants of childhood mortality.

Demographic Factors

These include sex, age, parity, and birth interval and as several studies, especially from the World Fertility Survey (see Preston 1985; Hobcraft, McDonald, and Rutstein 1985) have shown, all four have independent and synergistic (and in different situations, sometimes quite contradictory) effects on pregnancy outcome and child survival (for a recent summary of our knowledge in this area, see the review by the National Academy of Sciences 1989). Our results indicate several similar effects and undoubtedly partly explain the child mortality in our respondent households. However, their role in explaining regional differentials in child mortality is less clear, as discussed below. Moreover, the most interesting conclusion in this section is, as mentioned generally above, that it is often the case that cultural or socio-economic characteristics mediate in the relationship between a bio-demographic variable and child survival, rather than the bio-demographic variable being the intermediate factor which explains a socio-economic/cultural variable and child mortality relationship. The import of this statement will become clearer in the following paragraphs.

Sex

During the neonatal period, sex differentials in mortality in our study population are in the expected direction with girls having a relative advantage over boys. But after the first month of life, our two regional groups diverge greatly. In both cases girls lose their earlier advantage but for Tamil Nadu they now do the same as or only slightly worse than the boys, while for Uttar Pradesh male survival rates leave female children far behind. While the detailed sex pattern of infant and child mortality is discussed more fully in the next chapter, in the present context the important point is that the regional difference in the sex differential in child mortality is an important determinant of overall North–South differences in mortality in young children. That is, there is no common sex pattern of mortality which then accounts for regional differences in infant and child mortality through differences in the sex ratio of live births; instead it is the sex pattern of mortality itself which differs markedly in the two regional groups. Indeed, it is the much larger gap in female mortality between Tamil Nadu and Uttar Pradesh which explains a substantial part of the regional difference in overall child mortality; for boys the northern Indian disadvantage is nowhere near as hopeless.

Maternal Age and Parity

Our data find a very clear drop in the percentage of women who have lost a child as the mother's age at first live birth rises. For Uttar Pradesh, for instance, 69 per cent of the women who had their first live birth before the age of 15 had experienced some child loss. This percentage fell to 50 per cent and 44 per cent for women whose first delivery occurred at 18–19 years and 22–24 years respectively. But since the mean age at first live birth was 18.7 years for the Uttar Pradesh women and 18.4 years for the Tamil women, regional differentials in the proportion of women

Table. 5.3. Childhood mortality according to
maternal age at birth

Region and maternal age at birth	% children dead	% children dying within		% of total births occurring to mothers in this age-group
		1 year[a]	5 years[b]	
Uttar Pradesh (N=2458)				
15–19	38.0	20.4	12.8	2.0
20–24	33.4	22.4	8.0	24.9
25–29	26.5	15.7	8.0	35.4
30–34	19.4	10.9	8.8	22.7
35 +	17.0	10.0	5.8	15.1
Tamil Nadu (N=1998)				
15–19	27.5	20.0	5.0	2.0
20–24	24.6	15.7	7.1	29.5
25–29	21.6	11.5	8.1	36.0
30–34	22.8	11.2	8.8	20.2
35 +	24.0	12.0	9.3	12.4

[a] Excludes children born less than one year ago
[b] Excludes children born less than five years ago

who have lost a child are probably not due to differences in the initiation of childbearing.

Coming to more direct estimates of child mortality, Table 5.3 does indicate that children born to very young mothers are more likely to die, but does not really confirm the U-shaped relationship between maternal age at childbirth and child survival status found for 29 World Fertility Survey countries by Rutstein (1983). As expected, mortality falls with initial rises in mother's age, but for Uttar Pradesh at least, it surprisingly continues to fall even when the mother's age at delivery rises to enter the high-risk ages above 30 and even 35. However, results are also erratic for the 40 + age-group of mothers at birth for the WFS countries, so perhaps our results are not unique. While a part of this absence of a definite right arm to the U-shaped relation may be due to the relatively small number of events in the cells for the older maternal ages in most studies, in our study we feel that the continued downward trend in child mortality for older mothers is at least partly genuine. The reason is that the greater physical unsuitability of a birth at a late age is compensated somewhat by the better ability to raise a child with rising age, because of improved know-ledge about child-care with greater experience, more time and resources available for a child born at a later stage of the household life-cycle and, especially importantly, the greater potential for help from older children. With childbearing beginning around the age of 18, the typical infant with a 35-year-old mother is not going to be lacking in older siblings to act as a mother-substitute.

Indeed, in a multivariate analysis of World Fertility Survey data from 39 countries, Hobcraft, McDonald, and Rutstein (1985) found that when birth spacing was controlled, the apparent risks associated with older mothers were largely removed. And as Bongaarts (1987) has pointed out, other confounding factors may also be important, rendering spurious at least a part of the observed relation between maternal age at birth and child survival. For example, the effects on child mortality of increasing maternal age are the strongest in the overall low mortality countries. And in these countries births to older mothers occur mainly to women with high fertility; such women in turn belong to the lowest socio-economic population groups which have relatively high mortality.

However, for our Tamil sample, Table 5.3 does indicate more of the traditionally expected U-shaped curve for child survival by mother's age at birth (see col. 2), but once mortality is disaggre-gated by age, there are distinct and interesting differences from Uttar Pradesh. Infant mortality does first fall with rising age at delivery and then begins to rise again for mothers over 35, reflecting primarily biological factors. But mortality in early childhood (that is, in the 1–4 year age-group) actually rises with maternal age at delivery. We feel that the reason for this is the converse of the one that makes child mortality lower for older mothers in Uttar Pradesh, as discussed above. The older the Tamil woman, the greater the chance that she is employed outside the home; indeed the practice seems to be for women to spend the first few years of married life at home and then seek work, mainly in domestic service (for confirmation of this regional tendency, see Singh 1978). As we discuss in a later section, female employment levels are very distinctly positively associated with child mortality levels; we attribute this largely to the lower quality of child-care that a poor working mother is able to provide. This kind of reasoning probably also partly explains the fact that for Uttar Pradesh, mortality tends to fall with birth order, whereas for our Tamil sample, it instead rises steadily with birth order.

However, col. 5 of Table 5.3 suggests that maternal age at birth does not account for regional differentials in child survival. Although there are regional differences in maternal age at birth, these are in a direction favourable to both groups. Tamil Nadu has a smaller proportion of its births occurring to the higher-risk older women than does Uttar Pradesh. And conversely, Uttar Pradesh has a smaller proportion of its births occurring to the higher-risk younger women than does Tamil Nadu. While birth order may be connected either positively or negatively with mortality depending on the cultural group we are interested in, total fertility has a much less ambiguous relationship. For women of both regional groups, whatever their age, the child-loss experience is substantially greater for women whose fertility exceeds three live births (see Table 5.4). This is not a birth-order effect as already discussed, since higher fertility does not lead to higher mortality because of an excess of higher-order births: in high-fertility households, even earlier children have higher mortality.

Besides this unequivocal relationship, what is interesting is the regional difference in the extent of this relationship. For low-fertility women, Tamil Nadu shows lower child-loss experience than Uttar Pradesh; for higher-fertility women on the other hand, the Tamil experience of child mortality is even worse than the Uttar Pradesh one. Once more, we feel it is the child-care variable which mediates: the woman with more children is at a greater disadvantage if she works outside the home, as the Tamil mother is more likely to do. This probably also explains why for Uttar Pradesh the effect of parity is more or less similar if one looks at infant mortality or at mortality in early childhood; whereas for Tamil Nadu the risk of dying in infancy is 1.2 times greater for children born to mothers with a total of 4–6 as opposed to 1–3 live births, while it is 3.8 times greater for those dying in the 1–4 age-group in similar fertility categories, deaths in the 1–4 age-group being more a function of child-care quality rather than maternal depletion caused by several pregnancies.

Table 5.4. Distribution of women with at least one live birth according to their fertility and experience of child loss

| Age-group | Children ever born | Uttar Pradesh (N=573) | | Tamil Nadu (N=487) | |
		% of women who have lost a child	% women at this fertility level to total women in this age-group	% of women who have lost a child	% women at this fertility level to total women in this age-group
15–29	1–3	30.0	59.3	22.4	75.6
	4 +	66.4	40.7	72.6	25.4
30–49	1–3	34.3	24.1	24.4	35.2
	4 +	68.7	75.9	70.9	64.8

Birth Interval

In recent years there has been a great deal of research to indicate that even more pervasive and invidious than the other parental factors considered so far is the birth interval, both the one preceding and the one succeeding the index child (see Preston 1985; Gille 1985). Much of the evidence for this proposition is derived from analysis of World Fertility Survey data (see, for example, Rutstein 1983; Hobcraft, McDonald, and Rutstein 1983; Hobcraft, McDonald, and Rutstein 1985),[1] whereas from a survey of the earlier literature on the subject, Chen (1983) felt that the association between child mortality and birth intervals was inconclusive, mainly because of definitional and conceptual problems.

In the present study (see Table 5.5), a very clear negative association was found between deaths in childhood and the length of the succeeding as well as the preceding birth interval. This relationship persists in both regional groups, although it is slightly weaker for the South Indian women. The relationship is also stronger for the succeeding birth interval than it is for the preceding one, but this could be at least partly because of the reverse causation: higher child mortality rates lead to shorter subsequent birth intervals in the absence of contraception. But this direction of effect is not likely to be important in the case of mortality after infancy because the fertility suppressing effects of breast-feeding fall rapidly from this age. Yet we find that the 1–4 year death-rate also falls significantly with the length of the succeeding interval. This suggests that there is an important sibling competition effect, quite apart from a maternal depletion effect, which would focus on neonatal and infant mortality and which we are not able to disentangle from the reverse causality effect. In the case of the preceding birth interval, however, the intervening mechanism is likely to be maternal depletion rather than competition with other children (see Hobcraft, McDonald, and Rutstein 1985). The drain on her physical resources caused by a pregnancy following too soon after a live birth greatly reduces the survival prospects of the next child. Competition with the earlier sibling seems less important, especially when we consider that the mortality risks of short birth intervals are even greater if the previous child dies than when it survives.

At the same time, while it is true that socio-economic factors seem to be able to explain only a very small part of this strong

Table 5.5. Childhood mortality according to the length of the birth interval

A. Succeeding birth interval

Length of interval in months	% of children dead	% of children dying within						Age at death not stated	% births falling in this birth interval
		One week	1 month	1–11 months	1–4 years	One year	Five years		
Uttar Pradesh (N=1802)									
0–11	79.5	25.6	33.3	12.8	19.4	46.2	67.7	15.4	2.2
12–23	48.4	11.7	18.0	11.7	13.6	29.7	45.6	5.4	29.9
24–59	21.9	4.3	5.6	7.0	6.9	12.6	20.4	1.7	56.8
60 +	13.5	3.0	3.0	3.0	5.5	6.0	11.5	1.0	11.1
Tamil Nadu (N=1433)									
0–11	77.1	17.1	22.9	28.6	6.9	51.4	55.2	8.6	2.4
12–23	38.3	9.3	11.8	10.8	10.9	22.5	34.6	3.3	27.9
24–59	19.0	3.9	4.7	4.2	6.8	8.9	16.2	1.5	57.9
60 +	19.1	2.4	4.2	3.6	6.0	7.7	13.7	1.2	11.7

B. Preceding birth interval

Length of interval in months	% of children dead	% of children dying within						Age at death not stated	% births falling in this birth interval
		One week	1 month	1–11 months	1–4 years	One year	Five years		
Uttar Pradesh (N=1802)									
0–11	46.2	16.2	18.9	10.8	13.8	29.7	37.9	5.1	2.2
12–23	38.6	8.5	13.4	10.8	13.0	24.2	41.7	4.6	29.8
24–59	18.9	4.3	5.3	5.8	7.0	11.1	20.5	2.6	56.9
60 +	12.4	2.1	2.7	3.2	3.3	5.9	9.3	1.5	11.1
Tamil Nadu (N=1433)									
0–11	33.3	8.8	8.8	5.9	14.8	14.7	29.6	7.7	2.4
12–23	33.9	6.2	8.8	8.8	12.7	17.6	30.3	3.7	27.9
24–59	19.5	4.2	4.9	5.4	8.0	10.3	19.1	1.2	57.9
60 +	15.4	0.6	1.2	4.8	7.6	6.0	12.4	0.6	11.7

association, other factors may render spurious at least a part of the observed relation between child spacing and child mortality. For instance, Miller (1989) has concluded from an analysis of Hungarian and Swedish data that prematurity may be an important confounding variable in the observed sharp association between the length of the preceding birth interval and perinatal mortality.[2] Similarly, women with short inter-birth intervals may be also the women with worse child-care behaviour (for social or economic reasons), so that it is really the latter that explains their higher mortality experience. This kind of possibility increases the need, stressed at the beginning of this chapter, to identify high-risk women rather than merely high-risk attributes.

Coming back to the context of the present study, while the above findings have important implications for policies to reduce child death-rates, they seem to apply equally to both our cultural groups. As col. 10 of Table 5.5 indicates, there are no large cultural differences in the mean preceding and succeeding birth intervals for children belonging to the two cultural groups or in the distribution of intervals around these means. This implies that differences in birth intervals do not explain our regional differentials in infant and child mortality either. Nor does there seem to be any noticeable trend towards a shortening of birth intervals in the recent past. The mean succeeding birth interval does seem to be shorter for younger children but this is almost certainly because we exclude from our calculations last children, that is, those without a subsequent live birth, and in the younger age-groups these are naturally more such children that will in fact have a subsequent sibling; succeeding birth intervals for younger children are therefore biased towards shorter intervals. The preceding birth interval does not have this kind of bias and nor does it show any trend with birth cohort. This ties in with our other results which show no real tendency for the length of breast-feeding to have come down in recent times. And when it has, as in our South Indian working women, there seems to be a corresponding rise in contraceptive use.

Once again, this has considerable policy significance. While it is true that sterilization is the primary method of birth-control used in a country such as India, and that sterilization has many negative properties, the case for the promotion of temporary birth-control methods which follows is one which promotes temporary methods as a stopgap measure before the final irrevocable (in practice) sterilization decision is taken. This is important given the uncertainties of life in such a poor country setting. But it does not follow that temporary birth-control needs to be promoted to encourage longer intervals between births. As the National Academy of Sciences (1989) report concluded from a review of the available knowledge, the critical birth interval seems to be that below two years. There is no evidence that the gain in child survival is linearly related to birth intervals beyond this length.

The policy implication of the last paragraph is significant because it suggests a considerable narrowing of the target of a family-planning programme. By concentrating on women who have the desired (whether defined by themselves or by the state is a separate issue) number of children, the programme will use its resources more effectively than by forcing contraception on everyone exposed to intercourse.

To sum up, while all the usually implicated demographic factors do show the expected (and sometimes unexpected) relationships with child mortality in our study, only two of these seem possibly important determinants of regional differences in levels of child mortality. These two variables are sex and parity and they exert their influence in quite different ways. In the case of sex, while the sex distribution of births in the two groups is presumably similar (we discuss this further in the next chapter) the sex pattern of child mortality varies greatly in the two groups. In the case of fertility, the fertility impact on child mortality is similar for both groups, but the fertility levels themselves differ significantly in the two samples.

Environmental Contamination

This term, in Mosley and Chen's (1984) framework, refers to the transmission of infectious agents to children (and mothers). While the basic physical environment for both our cultural groups is the same, our results suggest that differences in regional household practices related to sanitation and hygiene lead to regional differences in the levels of potential exposure to disease, which are then reflected in regional differences in the actual incidence of illness.

Table 5.6 reports the overall mean number of illnesses recorded during the six-month longitudinal morbidity study for children from the two regional groups and the seasonal incidence of respiratory and gastro-intestinal complaints. The first finding is the lower incidence rates for the Tamil children, which are consistent with their lower mortality rates as well. This advantage can certainly not be attributed to their better nutritional status, except perhaps in the youngest age-group. Correct and complete immunization may also be partly responsible for exposure differences and, as discussed in the section on personal illness control, the Tamil children do have better immunization levels than those from Uttar Pradesh. However, immunization differences are not large and, in any case, immunization cannot explain the disaggregated picture of illness incidence evident in Table 5.6. To consider the relative Tamil advantage first, the greatest threat seems to be from the frailty of the physical shelters that go to make up the homes in this group. In our area, over 70 per cent of the Uttar Pradesh households have built a *pukka* (solid or cement) structure to house themselves, whereas less than half the South Indian families have been able to do so—not necessarily because of greater financial constraints, but also because of differing priorities. Given the severity of the Delhi winter, one wonders how much this greater exposure to the elements accounts for the higher level of respiratory illnesses in the Tamil children.

On the other hand, the disadvantage is towards the North Indian child in the case of gastro-intestinal ailments, and once more one must look for causes in the physical routes of transmission of this group of life-threatening illnesses. Contaminated food and water are the main sources of most intestinal infections and Black (1984) has stressed the role of sanitary waste disposal, avoidance of faecally contaminated water and objects, and the adoption of personal hygienic practices such as hand-washing, in controlling their spread. And on most of these counts, our sample households from Uttar Pradesh seem to do somewhat worse than those from Tamil Nadu. For example, while about 80 per cent of the South Indian households reported taking the trouble to throw their garbage in the official garbage heap in the colony (from where the Municipal vans are supposed to collect it regularly) the corresponding figure for Uttar Pradesh was only 67 per cent. The rest just dropped their rubbish outside the front door where it rots indefinitely either on the pavement or in the water drain which

Table 5.6. Regional differentials in the incidence of
illness in children

Region and age group	Mean number of illnesses in 6 months	Seasonal incidence of illness					
		Respiratory ailments (%)			Gastro-intestinal ailments (%)		
		Aug.	Oct.	Dec.	Aug.	Oct.	Dec.
Uttar Pradesh (N=882)							
< 1	3.2	6.0	14.8	9.6	17.0	11.3	10.6
1–4	2.9	6.7	11.5	12.0	12.5	7.9	2.6
5–9	1.8	4.9	7.9	6.3	2.7	3.0	2.5
All ages	2.4	5.8	10.3	9.1	8.5	6.2	3.7
Tamil Nadu (N=455)							
< 1	2.4	7.7	29.6	21.6	20.5	4.6	13.5
1–4	2.5	8.3	12.4	15.2	7.1	3.7	4.0
5–9	1.4	8.6	8.0	10.3	2.0	1.1	1.6
All ages	2.0	8.4	12.2	13.9	5.9	2.5	4.2

runs along each row of houses. The swarms of flies which collect on such exposed garbage cannot but be an important vehicle for gastro-intestinal ailments, especially as they flit between the garbage, the faeces in and around the public toilets and lanes, and the homes. One recalls clearly the all too familiar and depressing sight of young children periodically brushing away the flies which stubbornly settled on their bodies as they played outside their homes.

Then there is the natural spread of faecal contamination because of the relatively poor use of the public taps and toilets by the women and girls from Uttar Pradesh (for very young children, both regional groups keep away from the inconvenient public facilities available). For instance, even among girls aged 10–12 years, as many as 51 per cent use the space just outside the home for urinating; 25 per cent even defecate here. Admittedly, the Tamil girls' practices also leave much to be desired, but they are still better than their northern Indian counterparts, the corresponding figures for them being 36 per cent and 15 per cent. However, it would be misleading simply to put these high figures down to poor civic sense and hygiene. The embarrassment and insecurity felt in sending young girls to the public toilets provided by the local authorities are very strong, especially for the more conservative North Indian households, where women lead much more secluded lives, as has been discussed in various parts of this book. Indeed, this awkwardness and fear need to be a major consideration in the design of public facilities for such slum populations.

But custom and ignorance rather than shyness account for other differences in household practices detrimental to health. For example, only about 18 per cent of Uttar Pradesh households reported boiling the water given to babies, while for Tamil Nadu this figure was close to 30 per cent. This, especially coupled with the fact that about 84 per cent of the North Indian women delay the onset of breast-feeding for three or more days (this is 54 per cent for the Tamil women), during which time water constitutes an important ingredient of the baby's diet, means that the chances of neonatal infections are much greater for the North Indian babies.[3]

However, there is one potentially harmful domestic practice which differences in life-style cause to be more common for the Tamil women. This is the practice of storing cooked food for some time. Over a quarter of the households from Tamil Nadu reported that food is cooked in their homes only once a day, while for Uttar Pradesh close to 96 per cent of homes cooked their food afresh at every meal. Given the generally unsanitary environment, the heat in the summer, and the complete absence of food preservation devices such as refrigerators, one would expect a negative impact on the Tamil homes because of this household concession to working women, but Table 5.6 does not really find a higher incidence of gastro-intestinal illness in this group, so perhaps this is not as dangerous as it seems in theory.

Finally, a word about overcrowding as a factor in the morbidity and mortality of children. One can think of overcrowding differences at two levels—within the individual home and within a larger area composed of several households. At the individual household level, there is now a long-overdue interest in overcrowding as an intermediate variable in the observed link between fertility and child mortality in contemporary poor populations. For example, Aaby (1988) has hypothesized that such overcrowding leads to a greater intensity of exposure to infection and therefore higher case-fatality rates. This might also at least partly explain why, in the mid-nineteenth century, the crude death-rate in Glasgow was two and a half times as high for families living in one or two rooms, as compared to those in five or more rooms (Wrigley 1969).

At the community level, crowding cannot lead to regional differences in our sample groups, since they both occupy the same physical environment. A more appropriate comparison in this case is between urban and rural areas in the present study as well as in general. Consider the following statistics: according to the 1981 census, there were 57 households per square kilometre in rural Tamil Nadu and 55 in rural Uttar Pradesh; corresponding urban figures are 553 and 771. And in our urban slum we have a density of about 25 000 households in an area of about 815 hectares, that is, about 3000 households per square kilometre! Viewed in this light, the conclusion in Basu (1990) that the urban poor often have higher morbidity and mortality rates than rural populations seems all the more credible. In a similar but historical vein, Wrigley (1969) would attribute the higher urban mortality during the Industrial Revolution in Europe to the population density increases associated with urbanization rather than to industrialization *per se*. For example, the mortality in slums in large cities (which were more often commercial rather than industrial centres) was significantly higher than in industrial areas where people lived in relatively small villages and towns.

Nutrient Deficiency

Our data suggest that malnutrition is probably not a good explanation for regional differences in child mortality except in very specific and narrow ways, especially because, if anything, the South Indian children tend to score worse on this indicator than the children from Uttar Pradesh. For example, the mean length of breast-feeding is significantly lower for the Tamil children than it is for the children from Uttar Pradesh, as seen in Table 5.7.

Table 5.7. Mean length of breast-feeding (in months)

Number of months since birth	All live births		Only living children	
	Uttar Pradesh (N=1373)	Tamil Nadu (N=1003)	Uttar Pradesh (N=1106)	Tamil Nadu (N=824)
12–59	17.9	14.5	19.7	15.7
60–119	21.7	18.3	24.8	19.9
120–179	22.4	18.7	26.0	21.1
All ages	21.1	17.4	24.0	19.1

Note: Cases still breast-feeding have been excluded.

While we would attribute this regional differential to both convenience (a much larger proportion of the Tamil women work outside the home and therefore cannot indefinitely breast-feed their children) as well as to the greater modernization of the Tamil mothers (caused apparently by their higher levels of occupation outside the home, see Basu and Sundar 1988), it must be admitted that it is difficult to know how to interpret the connection of these breast-feeding differentials with final nutritional levels. For instance, it may well be that because of their earlier weaning, Tamil children get a more balanced diet than their North Indian counterparts. In our sample, the Tamil mothers reported starting their children on solids at an average age of 9.6 months, while the corresponding figure for Uttar Pradesh was 12.8 months.

But once solids have been introduced in both groups, the diet pattern for Tamil children does appear to be worse than for children for Uttar Pradesh. While practical reasons are certainly important, custom seems to be the main culprit for deleterious dietary practices.[4] Indeed, even in the states of origin, nutritional levels in Tamil Nadu are much worse than most other parts of the country (see Katona-Apte 1978; Gopalan *et al.* 1969). One important way in which such a differential occurs is through rice being the staple and sole cereal of the South Indian households, while the North Indians usually consume more than one cereal, together with a wide range of legumes and pulses. For example, in our longitudinal study only about 20 per cent of the Uttar Pradesh children aged 5–8 years reported having had just one kind of cereal on the previous day, while for Tamil Nadu, this figure was close to 80 per cent. In fact, from its all-India nutritional surveys, the National Institute of Nutrition (Gopalan and Raghavan 1969) has concluded that this regional difference in cereal consumption is linked to the regional patterns of severe protein–calorie malnutrition in the country, with levels being much higher in the predominantly rice-eating states of South India, West Bengal, and Orissa than in the rest of the country, where families generally eat two or more cereals and (especially) a variety of pulses and legumes. As discussed by Chakravarti (1982), poverty alone does not explain this pattern, since some areas where a multiplicity of cereals are eaten, such as Madhya Pradesh and eastern Uttar Pradesh, have similar, if not lower, standards of living to the areas where rice forms the bulk of the diet, leading to a poor intake of lysine and other essential amino acids. Even the greater level of non-vegetarianism in our Tamil sample[5] may be something of a disadvantage, because, given the high costs of non-vegetarian foods, too little of these are consumed and therefore much less protein obtained than among the predominantly vegetarian North Indians, who get their protein from much cheaper pulses.

But there are also a few ways in which the children of Tamil homes face better nutritional prospects than those from Uttar Pradesh, especially in the first few months of life. One important way is almost certainly the cultural difference in the initiation of breast-feeding. While the literature has devoted much attention to the importance of prolonged breast-feeding in both improving nutritional levels and reducing infection levels in children, much less has been said on the pernicious and probably peculiarly Indian practice of delaying the onset of breast-feeding until a few days after birth. The custom has become so entrenched that most women have not questioned its rationale enough to be able to answer any queries on the issue, beyond sometimes saying that colostrum is bad for the child. As Table 5.8 indicates, the majority of women in both our groups tend to delay the start of breastmilk until the third day after birth, but the women from Tamil Nadu seem to be more open to change in this regard: as many as 40 per cent of the younger women have accepted that breastmilk is good for the child from the very day of birth.

Table 5.8. Distribution of women according to
when they begin breast-feeding

% who begin breast-feeding	Uttar Pradesh (N=642)				Tamil Nadu (N=578)			
	Age-group				Age-group			
	< 30	30–49	50 +	All ages	< 30	30–49	50 +	All ages
Within one day of birth	9.6	6.2	0.0	7.6	39.9	36.8	30.4	37.7
On the second day of birth	6.7	9.2	21.7	8.4	8.1	13.4	0.0	10.7
On the third day or later	82.7	84.0	78.3	83.2	50.9	49.8	69.6	51.1

Besides impairing the nutritional status of young children, this custom is also probably partly responsible for the regional differentials in perinatal and neonatal mortality observed in Table 5.2, especially for births in the relatively distant past. The reason is not just the absence of protective antibodies in breast-milk but also the dangers inherent in the substitutes that are fed to the child if breastmilk is delayed: the two favourites are sugar-water and outside milk (that is, cow, buffalo, or goat milk). In both cases sterilization by boiling is usually far from adequate, quite apart from the poor digestibility of these foods. Another popular first feed is castor oil, as a purgative to clean out the stomach before breastmilk is begun.

Finally, there is the discrimination against children in the intra-household distribution of food. The deleterious effect of the common South Asian custom of women eating last, in a situation of limited resources, is well known. But where children are concerned, in our own study we found that only in a small percentage of cases (see Table 5.9) were children not among the first family members to be fed. However, there was also a regional difference in this and in households from the southern state of Tamil Nadu, children were given first preference in virtually all cases.

In spite of these two redeeming factors, on the balance it still appears that the Tamil children fare a little worse than those from Uttar Pradesh on overall achieved nutritional levels. As already mentioned in an earlier chapter, the present study included the taking of height and weight measurements of children below 12 years in the sample households. Height or reclining length was measured to the nearest 0.5 cm and weight to the nearest 0.2 kg.

Table 5.9. Eating order at the evening meal (%)

Region of origin	All eat together	Children eat first	Men eat first	Children and men eat first	No particular order
Uttar Pradesh (N=594)	44.8	21.2	8.4	11.8	13.8
Tamil Nadu (N=541)	76.7	5.4	1.1	1.3	15.5

Close to 88 per cent of the sample children had these anthropometric measurements recorded and we have no reason to
believe that the 12 per cent or so of children who could not be
measured constitute a biased sample in any way relevant to
the present context. The most frequent reason for not being
measured was physical unavailability for a few days at a stretch, so
that even repeated visits yielded no contact. Illness as a reason for
non-measurement occurred only in a handful of cases for both
regional groups. These anthropometric measurements were than
converted into nutritional levels using the sex-specific standards
of the US National Centre for Health Statistics (WHO 1983). The
following cut-off points were used for classification:

Weight-for-Age
  Normal/mild
    malnutrition   > o r = 80 per cent of standard
  Moderate
    malnutrition   = 60–79 per cent of standard
  Severe
    malnutrition   < 60 per cent of standard

Height-for-Age
  Normal/mild
    malnutrition   > o r = 95 per cent of standard
  Moderate
    malnutrition   = 85–94 per cent of standard
  Severe
    malnutrition   < 85 per cent of standard

Weight-for-Height
  Normal/mild
    malnutrition   > o r = 90 per cent of standard
  Moderate
    malnutrition   = 70–89 per cent of standard
  Severe
    malnutrition   < 70 per cent of standard

Height-for-age reflects chronic nutritional deprivation whereas
weight-for-age shows up both chronic and acute nutritional stress.
Both indices are age-dependent, so the accuracy of age-recording
is obviously an important determinant of results. In the present
study much effort was made to record correctly the ages of young

Table 5.10. Nutritional classification of children
according to weight-for-age (%)

Age in months	Uttar Pradesh (N=1149)			Tamil Nadu (N=745)		
	Normal/ mild malnu- trition	Moder- ate malnu- trition	Severe malnu- trition	Normal/ mild malnu- trition	Moderate malnu- trition	Severe malnu- trition
<11	49.1	36.2	14.6	61.1	34.7	4.1
12–23	34.0	53.6	12.3	37.1	48.7	14.1
24–59	41.1	50.0	8.8	40.7	50.2	9.0
60–119	39.0	54.0	6.9	30.5	58.6	10.7
120–143	24.5	57.5	17.9	12.0	62.9	25.0
All ages	37.5	51.7	10.7	34.2	53.6	12.0

children through a series of internal cross-checks in the questionnaire and through extensive instructions to field staff about locally
suitable probes and about not accepting ages rounded off to the
nearest complete figure. We believe that the resulting record of
ages is fairly correct (that is, as correct as is possible in the absence
of birth registration and in a culture where exact age is not a
relevant concept), but we also support our results with nutritional
classification by the age-independent weight-for-height criterion,
although this index has its limitations (see Chen, Chowdhury, and
Huffman 1980).

The results are set out in Tables 5.10 and 5.11 below. Height-
for-age gave very similar results to weight-for-age and is therefore
not presented. By both the weight-for-age and height-for-age
criteria, in the first year of life the level of severe malnutrition is
higher for Uttar Pradesh than for Tamil Nadu, but beyond the age
of one, the South Indian children do considerably worse than
their North Indian counterparts. This fits in with the better
antenatal care, the earlier start of breast-feeding, and the earlier
weaning in our Tamil sample, which then give way to worse
dietary habits in slightly older children.

So the finding is that severe malnutrition is greater in the Tamil
Nadu sample than in that from Uttar Pradesh. And yet, as Tables
5.1 and 5.2 showed, infant and child mortality are distinctly lower

Table 5.11. Nutritional classification of children
according to weight-for-height (%)

Age in months	Uttar Pradesh (N=1119)			Tamil Nadu (N=703)		
	Normal/ mild malnu- trition	Moder- ate malnu- trition	Severe malnu- trition	Normal/ mild malnu- trition	Moderate malnu- trition	Severe malnu- trition
<11	69.8	18.8	11.3	62.3	27.5	10.1
12–23	50.0	42.7	7.2	60.8	29.7	9.4
24–59	60.7	34.8	4.4	63.1	32.6	4.2
60–119	51.0	44.5	4.3	55.9	40.6	3.3
120–143	55.0	43.5	1.4	47.0	48.0	4.9
All ages	56.0	39.2	4.7	57.7	37.1	5.1

in the former group. Our result is a clear deviation from the generally expected relationship between malnutrition and mortality. But why is there such an expected relationship? Intuitively it seems obvious that greater malnutrition should mean more deaths, but this is at least partly because one's intuition tends to confuse malnutrition and starvation. The latter certainly does lead to death, but even with a more sophisticated definition of malnutrition, while one may accept that theoretically and *ceteris paribus* the risk of death increases with greater malnutrition, the fact of the matter is that in the real world all other things are not equal, so that when one examines the actual evidence it is seen that, except in a limited number of cases, changes in mortality over time or cross-sectional differentials in mortality are not really explained by secular changes or cross-sectional differentials in nutritional levels. This is particularly so when one is looking at differences within otherwise homogeneous groups (as opposed to differences between such groups).

The absence of an obvious and general malnutrition–mortality link has been discussed in detail elsewhere (see Basu 1989), but it is worth mentioning here that it also seems to be agreed in the literature that one aspect of health which is not affected by malnutrition is the incidence or frequency of occurrence of infections (Scrimshaw, Taylor, and Gordon 1968; Chen, Huq, and D'Souza 1981; Koenig and D'Souza 1986). And our own data, while admittedly less specialist than those on which this result is generally based, also support such a conclusion. The only relationship that the incidence rates of illness seen in Table 5.6 seem to show with malnutrition is that of the strong falling ill more often than the weak. But this is absurd of course (unless by the strong we mean the obese, but obesity was not a confounding factor in our generally deprived slum population) and the more plausible interpretation is probably that, as in the case of mortality, morbidity too seems overall to be unrelated to nutritional status in today's circumstances, other determinants of exposure to illness being of greater importance.

Injury

No significant differences were found between the two groups in the incidence of accidents and injuries either as causes of death in the retrospective data or as causes of ill health or debilitation during the longitudinal study. If anything, the Tamil children had a slightly higher proportion dying from accidental causes than their North Indian counterparts. But given the somewhat unsatisfactory nature of our cause-of-death retrospective data and the small absolute numbers of cases reported under accidents and injuries, we would not lay much store by these results.

Personal Illness Control

This is the last category of proximate determinant in Mosley and Chen's (1984) framework and our evidence suggests that in the context of regional differentials in overall childhood mortality (as distinct from sex-specific childhood mortality which is discussed in the next chapter) it is important in very specific ways. This variable includes behaviours which prevent as well as cure disease states. Our results indicate that regional background operates through the former group of behaviours to influence mortality, while in the case of the use of curative (especially modern) medical care, the primary determinant of cultural differentials is the availability of services rather than the willingness to use them. However, there are some interesting differences in the domestic handling of illness episodes.

To begin with prophylactic immunizations, cols. 3 and 4 of Table 5.12 indicate that the Uttar Pradesh mother is, if anything, more likely to have her children immunized than her Tamil counterpart. And for both these groups, overall immunization levels are astonishingly high. However, it should be noted that the immunization status of living children may not correctly reflect the presence or absence of regional differences, because such differences may be drowned in regional differences in mortality. But Table 5.12 indicates that even when all live births are considered, although percentages immunized are now lower for both groups, there are no major regional differentials.

But these data are somewhat misleading, since the catch-all term of 'any immunization' includes, at least for the older children who show such excellent rates of compliance, the smallpox vaccination which was compulsory when they were born. And when we look at a more relevant and specific immunization such as the triple antigen (as is done in rows 3 and 4; note that the same findings apply to the polio and BCG vaccines), we are very far from the universal vaccination levels which UNICEF would have had us reach by 1990. This same kind of deception is likely when one looks at secondary data from the region of origin. For example, the Registrar General of India's (1981*a*) survey of infant and child mortality found no major differences in the percentages of rural children aged 5 who had received any immunization as indicated in the first row of Table 5.13. But, as the following

Table 5.12. Regional differentials in the immunization status of children

| Immunizations received (%) | Uttar Pradesh | | Tamil Nadu | |
| | Age-group (years) | | | |
	1–4	5–9	1–4	5–9
All live births:				
any immunizations	74.0	68.7	70.3	71.0
Only living children:				
any immunizations	83.2	82.8	77.3	81.5
at least one dose of triple antigen	59.7	48.7	45.2	40.6
all three doses of triple antigen	16.6	14.2	27.8	27.6

Sample size. Uttar Pradesh—1114 live births, 887 living children; Tamil Nadu—777 live births, 629 living children.

Table 5.13. Immunization status of children aged 5 years in Uttar Pradesh and Tamil Nadu

| Immunizations received (%) | Uttar Pradesh | | | | Tamil Nadu | | | |
| | Rural | | Urban | | Rural | | Urban | |
	Male	Female	Male	Female	Male	Female	Male	Female
Any immunization	93.0	92.0	94.8	94.9	99.5	99.3	97.8	99.0
Smallpox	91.7	90.0	91.6	92.6	95.5	95.2	91.1	92.6
Triple antigen	2.5	2.5	19.6	22.5	15.6	15.1	43.8	40.2
BCG	15.8	16.1	42.3	44.7	45.1	46.1	68.8	66.3
Polio	15.8	0.0	6.2	6.8	2.0	2.2	10.2	10.1

Source: Registrar General of India (1981), *Survey of Infant and Child Mortality, 1979*, Government of India, New Delhi.

rows of this table subsequently indicate, it is again smallpox which is the great equalizer. Where triple antigen, polio and BCG are concerned, there is a yawning gap between the two states and once more, for both states, levels of protection are disappointing.

But in our sample, where services are controlled, the North Indian child still does slightly better than the South Indian even when one looks at specific kinds of immunization (see, for example, row 3 of Table 5.12). Where then is the important cultural difference? The difference lies in perseverance and in the extent of the sharp fall in the numbers of children who are allowed to take the full recommended course of three doses of vaccine (see the two bottom rows of Table 5.12). This stresses once again the social constraints to effective vaccine use discussed by Mosley (1984). Our field information suggested that the woman from Uttar Pradesh was much more alarmed by the presence of the adverse side-effects of immunization than was her Tamil Nadu counterpart who, for various reasons, was more difficult to contact for the first dose of vaccine but who, once contacted, did not recoil as vehemently from the fever which resulted in a vaccinated child. This was the situation in our urban slum environment, with relatively good access to health services and relatively high access to outside information. In the absence of these, one wonders what continuation rates would have looked like in the rural areas, if they had been available to complement Table 5.13, especially for Uttar Pradesh.

There is one more area where there are important cultural differentials in the use of preventive medical care: the area of childbirth. According to the 1979 survey of infant and child mortality (Registrar General of India 1981 *a*), fully 94 per cent of rural Uttar Pradesh births had been delivered by untrained personnel while in rural Tamil Nadu the figure was 50 per cent. This differential is not explained by accessibility alone, as is clear from Table 5.14 based on our survey data. Even for the births which occurred in Delhi and which therefore theoretically faced the same institutional choices, the Uttar Pradesh sample clings to the home as the best locale for a delivery, though admittedly the hospital stands a better chance than it does in the region of origin. For Tamil Nadu on the other hand, births in Delhi are three times more likely than those for the Uttar Pradesh group to have occurred in a hospital.[6]

Table 5.14. Distribution of all live births according to place of birth and institution of delivery

A. Uttar Pradesh (N=2376)

Place of birth

Institution of delivery	Uttar Pradesh					Delhi				
	Years since birth					Years since birth				
	< 5	5–9	10–14	15 +	All ages	< 5	5–9	10–14	15 +	All ages
Home	96.8	96.2	99.2	99.3	98.4	87.0	91.6	90.5	85.7	88.8
Hospital	3.3	3.3	0.8	0.4	1.5	12.6	8.4	9.5	11.8	10.7
Other/NS	0.0	0.5	0.0	0.2	0.2	0.4	0.0	0.0	2.5	0.5

B. Tamil Nadu (N=1921)

Place of birth

Institution of delivery	Tamil Nadu					Delhi				
	Years since birth					Years since birth				
	< 5	5–9	10–14	15 +	All ages	< 5	5–9	10–14	15 +	All ages
Home	45.3	53.2	70.5	74.8	70.5	67.7	63.4	48.0	55.0	60.3
Hospital	54.7	46.8	29.5	25.0	29.4	32.3	36.7	52.0	44.5	39.6
Other/NS	0.0	0.0	0.0	0.2	0.1	0.0	0.0	0.0	0.5	0.1

Even more interesting is the nature of the assistance received during delivery by the two groups as shown in Table 5.15. The paramedical health-worker occupies a disappointingly low place in all cases: the women will only accept the two extremes, either a trained doctor or an untrained though often experienced neighbourhood helper. The great reliance on the traditional birth attendant or *dai* is expected, given the large numbers of home deliveries. What is surprising is the frequency with which the friend, neighbour, or relative comes to the rescue, even among the most recent births. While this is a positive reflection of the informal networks of help and co-operation which the women, especially from Uttar Pradesh, have built up in the city, it does not speak too well of the persuasive powers of the existing health services, not just in ensuring a hygienic delivery but also in providing much needed antenatal care. In fact we found it to be the case that even for hospital deliveries, the registration at the maternity centre or hospital and subsequent antenatal check-ups began at an extremely late stage of the pregnancy and were usually done only because such prior registration is required if a woman in labour is to gain admittance.

What explains the Uttar Pradesh woman's greater reluctance to have a hospital delivery? The first and dominant reason appeared to be fear. It is one thing to visit a doctor for a child's ailment, but quite another to subject oneself to a few days and nights in what is perceived to be an essentially unfamiliar and often hostile environment. Greer's (1984) analysis of hospital-based childbirth is probably particularly relevant to the poor, un-educated slum-dweller from a village and deserves an extensive quote:

removing the woman from her own territory to the unfamiliar environ-ment of the hospital has a frightening and disorienting effect which is intensified by the further insistence on moving her from place to place once labour is well under way. Instead of being aided by familiar figures whom she trusts, who have nothing else to do for the time being but assist her, she is competing for the attention of professionals, who will not give her their undivided attention unless she earns it by turning into a medical emergency (Greer 1984).

These observations are particularly valid for our North Indian sample who have a very limited exposure to the outside world, who have been brought up in an area of extremely limited health

Table 5.15. Distribution of all live births according to help received by mother during delivery

| | Uttar Pradesh (N=2482) | | | | | Tamil Nadu (N=2007) | | | | |
| | Years since birth | | | | | Years since birth | | | | |
	< 5	5–9	10–14	15 +	All ages	< 5	5–9	10–14	15 +	All ages
Doctor	11.1	7.5	7.7	4.5	7.7	38.8	39.6	44.0	30.5	36.6
Health worker	3.0	2.3	4.2	2.0	2.8	2.1	1.9	1.7	1.3	1.6
Dai[a]	50.9	46.0	43.9	36.3	44.0	45.3	38.9	35.4	40.5	48.3
Friend/relative/neighbour	29.5	38.1	39.3	48.2	39.0	12.2	17.7	16.9	21.4	17.8

[a] Local midwife.

Note. The percentages do not add up to 100 because of a few cases which belong to the 'others', 'no-one' and 'not stated' categories.

services and who belong to a tradition of much less female autonomy than their South Indian counterparts (see Chapter 3). To their subsequent mistrust of a hospital-based delivery must be added two very real fears which were repeatedly expressed: the fear that they would be forcibly sterilized after the delivery and the fear that the baby born to them (especially if it were male) would be exchanged for a worse (generally female) one from a more influential mother. While the latter fear is largely imaginary[7] one cannot say the same about the former with a government health and family-planning programme which is justifiably proud, in terms of sheer numbers, of its record of post-partum sterilizations.

Finally, there is the sheer physical inconvenience of a hospital delivery. Though such a delivery is theoretically free of charge, the actual costs incurred can be enormous. There is the expense of transport to the hospital (often more than once), the need to find efficient help not just to run the home but also to make the daily trips to the hospital with food and other necessities for the new mother, and the time and expense involved in getting registered for a hospital birth.

All these disadvantages often mean that a woman has to be very strongly motivated before she accepts a hospital-based childbirth and unfortunately often the only motivation strong enough is one derived from sudden complications of pregnancy or delivery. While it is true that the medical risks of a home delivery in a poor country are higher than a hospital one, under present circumstances, the policy prescription which follows should probably be one which greatly improves the domiciliary (especially antenatal) services for delivery instead of a blanket attempt to increase hospital births.

How does the institution of delivery affect child survival? In a state-level analysis of infant mortality in India, Jain (1985) concluded that the percentage of births attended by trained medical practitioners explained a high proportion of the regional variations in infant mortality and that this was also one of the main variables through which the non-medical variable of female literacy operated. In our own survey, the hospital delivery turns out to be more successful in ensuring that a child lives beyond a week than a delivery which is conducted at home, but for the Uttar Pradesh sample at least, the difference is probably larger than it appears because several of the (already few) hospital births (especially in the relatively distant past) are to women who resort to the hospital only in an emergency. That is, there is not a random allocation of births between the home and the hospital, the latter get an undue proportion of high-risk cases. But this trend is changing and an increasing overall tendency for women to have a hospital birth is probably reflected in the higher mortality of home births for the recent past. The role of the hospital is larger when one compares mothers who had received some antenatal medical care during their last pregnancy with those who had received no such care: for both regional groups the proportion of surviving children is appreciably higher in the former case. And since as many as 46 per cent of the Tamil women reported having received some antenatal care during the last pregnancy, as compared to 34 per cent of the Uttar Pradesh women (these differences would be even larger for the earlier births), this probably accounts for at least some of the regional differential in infant (especially neonatal) mortality.

To these medical interventions sought for chidbirth must be added the cultural beliefs and practices which accompany any pregnancy. For example, as many as 65 per cent of the North Indian women and 38 per cent of the South Indian women reported that they had reduced their food intake during their last pregnancy. The belief appeared to be that such nutritional restraint would result in an easier delivery. The regional contrast was even sharper in the case of women who actually ate more than usual during the pregnancy—5 per cent for Uttar Pradesh and 30 per cent for Tamil Nadu. The remaining women in both groups continued as usual, with not even the occasional indulgence of some special food during the pregnant state.

So much for preventive illness control. Coming to modern curative medical care, our data indicate that although there are interesting intra-household differentials in use (especially by sex, as discussed in the next chapter), once access to services is controlled, cultural background is not a serious bar to their overall utilization.[8] It is true that the Registrar General of India's survey of infant and child mortality (1981*a*) found that in rural Uttar Pradesh only about 34 per cent of infant deaths and 59 per cent of deaths of children aged 1–4 years had been attended by a trained medical practitioner, while in rural Tamil Nadu the corresponding figures were 61 per cent and 64 per cent. But our

data indicate that this regional difference is better explained
by the fact that by the end of 1984, Uttar Pradesh had one doctor
per 13 000 population and one hospital bed per 43 000 rural
population, the corresponding numbers for Tamil Nadu being
8000 and 12 000 respectively (Department of Health and Family
Welfare 1985).

To illustrate this more vividly, Table 5.16 presents our data on
regional similarities and differences in the medical handling of
four of the most commonly occurring group of illnesses during
the six-month longitudinal morbidity study in which children
below the age of 12 were visited once in two weeks. The illness groups are undefined fevers, respiratory ailments, gastro-
intestinal ailments, and skin problems. While it is true that these
are very general categories and can include a range of conditions
from the mild to the severe, we have reason to believe that there
are no significant differences in the pattern of this range between
the two groups. Moreover, a fairly intense effort was made by the
field staff during the longitudinal study to keep a tab on the outcome of illness states which had been noted during previous visits
and to physically satisfy themselves about the reliability of illness
reporting by mothers.

The first and most striking finding of Table 5.16 is the over-
whelming faith in modern or Western-type medicine, whatever
the regional origin, nature of illness, or age of the sufferer. This
faith seems to remain unshaken however backward the household
in other respects, with the uneducated or the lower castes often
even more eager to seek what they perceive as qualified allopathic
help than their socio-economic superiors. Nor is this finding
unique to the present study. Several writers (for example, Banerjee 1973; Lieban 1977; Caldwell, Reddy, and Caldwell 1983) have
described the strong faith in modern medicine which often exists
simultaneously with traditional or supernatural beliefs about
disease causation. Perhaps Erasmus (1961) was quite right in stressing that 'even uneducated and illiterate people are not simple
tradition bound puppets of their culture. Given adequate opportunity to measure the advantages of a new alternative, they act to
maximize their expectations.'

Whatever its other faults, the ability of modern clinical medicine
to eliminate the symptoms of ill-health and even ward off death,
at least in the short run, is easily demonstrable (and has been

demonstrated, for example, in case-studies of China, Kerala, Sri Lanka, and Costa Rica; see Halstead, Walsh, and Warren 1985). It appeared to be well demonstrated to our sample households as well and their touching belief in the antibiotic, especially if it came in injection form (for a review of the excessive popularity of the injection in most of the Third World, see Wyatt 1984) was in sharp contrast to their fear and mistrust of preventive vaccinations. The logic behind this anomalous attitude could not be easily faulted, after all they could plainly see how curative medicine got rid of the symptoms of ill-health while immunization actually produced such symptoms in a normally healthy child.

Regional differentials in the use of modern curative medicine are therefore revealing by their absence. But even more interesting than the unalloyed faith in modern medicine is the kind of medical practitioner that is favoured. Our data (see Table 5.16) indicate a uniform tendency to consider the private practitioner to be superior to the government one, even though the services of the latter are free. The reasons for this are complex and include the much longer wait for attention at the government clinic, the greater impersonality of the government clinic, and, very importantly, the human inclination to devalue what is free. But perhaps most relevant of all is the fact that the private practitioner (it would be inaccurate to call him the private doctor as several of these individuals do not have a formal medical qualification), like his clients, believes in quick results. So he usually does not even have a separate consultation fee—what he charges instead is a flat rate of something like Rs 5 for a consultation and an injection, even before he has diagnosed the illness. Such indiscriminate use of drugs is less common in the government dispensary because there is some attempt to avoid unnecessary medication and also because the government dispensary is chronically short of drugs.

How does cultural origin affect the choice of medical practitioner? Although the bulk of the preference in both groups is for the private doctor, this preference is somewhat stronger in the Tamil group. But we feel that this is related to the life-style differences between the two groups rather than to any intrinsic cultural factors. As the women from Tamil Nadu are much more likely to be employed than those from Uttar Pradesh and as most of the government health facilities function during the daytime (usually in the later morning), the working woman is forced to

Table 5.16. The handling of children's illness episodes according to region of origin, type of illness, and age

A. Uttar Pradesh

Nature of illness	Age-group (in years)	No treatment	Govern-ment doctor	Private doctor	Home remedy (modern)	Home remedy (tradi-tional)	Others	Mean no. of treatments per treated illness	Of all cases seen by doctor, % seen by private doctor
(1)	(2)	(3)	(4)	(5)	(6)	(7)	(8)	(9)	(10)
Fever	< 1	8.3	15.0	83.3	6.7		1.1	1.15	84.7
	1–4	5.5	25.3	76.4	2.2	1.1	1.5	1.12	75.1
	5–9	9.0	20.3	77.4	2.3			1.12	79.2
	10–11	11.5	21.3	70.5	1.6			1.06	76.8
	All ages	7.8	21.8	76.8	2.8	0.5	0.9	1.11	77.9
Respiratory illness	< 1	20.8	17.7	59.4	8.3	1.0	1.0	1.11	77.0
	1–4	18.3	12.5	66.1	4.0	1.8	3.1	1.07	84.1
	5–9	16.2	14.4	65.3	8.4	1.8	1.2	1.09	82.0
	10–11	20.3	20.3	50.0	10.9	1.6	6.3	1.12	71.1
	All ages	18.3	14.9	62.8	6.9	1.6	2.5	1.09	80.8
Gastro-intestinal illness	< 1	15.8	14.9	73.7	2.6	3.5	0.9	1.14	83.2
	1–4	13.4	19.3	73.8	1.5	1.5	1.5	1.13	79.3
	5–9	16.2	17.6	67.6	1.4	5.4	2.7	1.13	79.4
	10–11	25.0	12.5	68.8				1.08	84.6
	All ages	15.0	17.5	72.4	1.7	2.7	1.5	1.13	80.5
Skin disease	< 1	10.0	33.3	66.7	6.7	3.3		1.22	66.7
	1–4	23.3	16.3	55.8	7.8	3.1	0.8	1.09	77.4
	5–9	15.1	26.1	59.7	5.9	5.0	0.8	1.15	69.6
	10–11	19.2	23.4	48.9	8.5	2.1		1.05	67.7
	All ages	18.5	22.5	57.2	7.1	3.7	0.6	1.12	61.4

B. Tamil Nadu

Nature of illness	Age-group (in years)	% receiving the following treatment						Mean no. of treatments per treated illness	Of all cases seen by doctor, % seen by private doctor
		No treatment	Government doctor	Private doctor	Home remedy (modern)	Home remedy (traditional)	Others		
(1)	(2)	(3)	(4)	(5)	(6)	(7)	(8)	(9)	(10)
Fever	< 1	10.0	10.0	80.0				1.00	88.9
	1–4	9.7	9.7	77.4	6.5		3.2	1.04	88.9
	5–9	14.8	14.8	57.4	14.8			1.02	79.6
	10–11	10.5	5.3	73.7	10.5			1.00	93.3
	All ages	14.4	13.1	65.4	9.8		0.7	1.03	83.3
Respiratory illness	< 1	15.7	9.8	76.5				1.02	88.6
	1–4	16.3	9.3	71.3	5.4	1.6		1.05	88.5
	5–9	26.3	10.0	47.5	17.5			1.02	82.6
	10–11	23.5	17.7	47.1	11.8			1.00	72.7
	All ages	19.5	10.1	63.9	8.3	0.7		1.03	86.2
Gastro-intestinal illness	< 1	18.4	13.2	73.7		5.3		1.13	84.8
	1–4	15.3	23.7	64.4	1.7			1.06	73.1
	5–9	14.3	14.3	57.1	14.3			1.00	80.0
	10–11	25.0		75.0				1.00	100.0
	All ages	16.7	18.5	67.6	1.9			1.08	78.5
Skin disease	< 1			100.0				1.00	100.0
	1–4	15.2	15.2	63.0	6.5	2.2		1.03	80.6
	5–9	12.1		66.7	12.1	9.1		1.00	100.0
	10–11	50.0		50.0				1.00	100.0
	All ages	14.6	7.9	66.3	7.9	4.5		1.01	89.4

seek the services of a more conveniently open private practitioner. However, since even in Tamil Nadu itself women's employment levels are much higher than in Uttar Pradesh, this question of convenient timings remains relevant while designing health services for South Indian groups in general. In fact, this probably partly explains why an all-India study by the National Council of Applied Economic Research (NCAER 1985) in Delhi found that the per capita expenditure both on medical care and on medicines in low-income groups in both urban and rural areas were higher for households in South India than for those in North India.

Once modern clinical medicines have been considered, the residual kinds of treatment (of which 'no treatment' forms an essential and relevant category) are best examined by disaggregating illnesses according to symptomatic type. To begin with, for both regions and all age-groups, 'no treatment' is much lower for fevers than for respiratory or gastro-intestinal problems as is evident in Table 5.16. Our qualitative information indicates that this is a partly a reflection of an undefined fever causing greater panic than a clearer symptom like a cough or diarrhoea which is seen as irritating but not incapacitating in the same way as a fever. In fact, respiratory and gastro-intestinal ailments are accepted as an inevitable part of life because of their greater frequency and this very frequency make them appear less threatening to life or well-being. The second reason for the alacrity with which fevers are treated is that they are seen to be much more easily cured by modern medicine; naturally, since an anti-pyretic is the easiest and most effective medicine to prescribe and to take, and, because it is relatively safe, doctors have no qualms about recommending it. The greater importance given to fever and the greater efficiency of the resulting treatment is also evident in the much lower mean durations of episodes of fever than of respiratory or gastro-intestinal complaints: for example, among 5–9-year-old boys from Uttar Pradesh the average durations of an episode of fever, respiratory infection, and gastro-intestinal infection were 7.5 days, 9.8 days, and 16.7 days respectively.

Regional patterns are as expected. In the same logical vein as above, the more tradition-bound and secluded Uttar Pradesh mother is not only more likely to treat fever than respiratory or gastro-intestinal problems, she is also much more likely to treat fever than the Tamil mother and at the same time much less likely to treat the latter ailments than is her Tamil counterpart. This is in line with her greater tendency to treat these more frequent illnesses as more inevitable or fate-ordained and therefore less amenable to intervention.

The greater self-confidence of the Tamil households is also apparent in the much greater ease with which they resort to self-medication with modern drugs than do their North Indian counterparts. This is the case for all illnesses in general but especially for fevers and respiratory complaints. That they are well prepared for such home treatment is seen in the fact that about 25 per cent of the Tamil households reported keeping pain-killers at home and close to 32 per cent kept at least one kind of modern medicine, while for Uttar Pradesh the corresponding percentages were 14 and 25 respectively. In fact even a study in rural Tamil Nadu (Rao and Richard 1984) reported that as many as 70 per cent of households preferred self-treatment with allopathic medicines for common ailments at the initial stages of a disease.

Such confidence in one's ability to handle illnesses oneself may be misplaced and even dangerous, but even more worrying is the finding that the only group for which the Uttar Pradesh households are more likely to try modern home remedies more frequently than the Tamil ones is the highly vulnerable group of children below the age of 1, whatever the category of illness. Fortunately, the Tamil sample tends to leave this age-group strictly out of its household medical practice experiments. But even more disturbing is the finding that for both groups, infants are much more likely to be untreated for an illness than children over 1; infancy is the most vulnerable stage of life and yet infant illnesses are more likely to be left alone. However, it would be misleading to equate this with an uncaring attitude to such illnesses. On the contrary, to quote Caldwell, Reddy, and Caldwell (1983), 'Both a casualness about the conditions of birth and a lack of intensive care during infancy denote, in fact, a high degree of concern. Any obvious trouble about the child or any precautions against sickness would invite the jealousy of demons and may well result in the death of the child.' However, it is worth noting that for Uttar Pradesh, in the case of fever, the relatively low treatment rates for infants mask a strong sex differential: male infants are much more likely than children of other ages of both sexes to be treated for fever. This is in line with the general panic caused by fever plus the strong male preference in the North Indian sample. Both these together are compelling enough to overcome the fatalistic attitude which is generally adopted towards illness in young children. Finally, for both groups, skin problems are relatively more likely to receive modern home treatment (usually some kind of ointment) than are other illnesses.

The converse of the Tamil households' greater faith in home medication with modern drugs is the Uttar Pradesh sample's relatively greater resort to traditional home remedies and 'other' or non-allopathic forms of treatment, especially for coughs, colds, and diarrhoea. However, this often involves the use of the more traditional kinds of treatment prior to, subsequent to, or sometimes simultaneously with modern Western treatment. This explains our finding that the mean number of treatments per treated illness is consistently higher for Uttar Pradesh than it is for Tamil Nadu. Such plurality of treatment has been noted by others (for example, Caldwell, Reddy, and Caldwell 1983) and seems to be a regular intermediate stage in the move towards more or less complete dependence on Western medicine (or Western medicines; as Alland (1970) has pointed out, the major interest is in modern drugs, not really in overall modern methods of handling illness).

Finally, we have the role of traditional beliefs about disease which are often harmful. While it is true that once the worth of a medical treatment has been clearly demonstrated, it is possible for its use to coexist with a continued belief in the supernatural or otherwise traditional origins of a disease, it is sometimes the case that the latter beliefs are strong enough to resist any such demonstration about the value of professional help. I illustrate this with an anecdote: during a part of our longitudinal study, there was a minor epidemic of chickenpox in the area. The first surprising thing was that this was always reported as smallpox (in fact even some of our interviewers had difficulties in appreciating that these are two separate diseases). This was because smallpox, chickenpox, and even measles were perceived not as separately classified illnesses but as a condition of being visited by a particular goddess—*Mariamma* for the South Indians and *Sitala* for the North Indians. Indeed the Tamil word for the disease, *amman valayadukiral*, roughly translates as 'the goddess is playing'. Such divine visits are not to be interfered with and the general policy appeared to be one of seeking absolutely no medical help even to ward off secondary infections. During an episode of chickenpox all the taboos of a temple were maintained: no menstruating woman went near the affected child, sexual abstinence was practised in the household, and, most forceful of all, if a child died (as some did during our study) no tears were shed.

Similarly, even non-supernatural beliefs about illness and optimum treatment may turn out to be misplaced. What is troubling is that the modern health-care system, both governmental and privately operated, has been so successfully and fully involved in its curative and to some extent immunization roles that it seems to have made no attempt to influence potentially dangerous traditional beliefs. For example, a large number of our respondents continue to believe that breast-feeding should not be commenced until the third day after delivery and that food and water should be drastically curtailed during a bout of diarrhoea. Such views and beliefs exist in both our regional groups but more so in the North Indian women, and are a negative commentary on the role of the health-care apparatus in education and information.

5.3. Socio-Economic Influences on Child Mortality

The earlier section has discussed the possible proximate determinants of our observed regional differentials in childhood mortality. One of the striking findings there was the need to specify the population under study before defining a proximate determinant–child mortality relationship, even in the case of the supposedly biological proximate determinants such as sex and maternal age. That is, cultural background has an important influence on the nature of the effect of proximate or intermediate variables on survival chances. It is therefore no longer surprising to find that socio-economic variables too are often related to childhood mortality levels in quite different ways in different population groups. We illustrate this in greater detail with the variable of mother's education. We also briefly consider a surprising relationship between child mortality and maternal work status.

Maternal Education

It was Caldwell (1979) who first convincingly demonstrated with field data from Ibadan, Nigeria that maternal education is a more important determinant of child survival than virtually any other socio-economic characteristic. This conclusion has since then been drawn so religiously by so many studies that by now it appears rather banal. However, we still add our findings to the pool.

As expected, the main result in the first row of Table 5.17 indicates that educated mothers experience fewer child deaths than uneducated mothers. But what is more interesting is the regional differential in the extent of the maternal education–child mortality link, and the age at death pattern of the relationship. To begin with regional differentials, Table 5.17 suggests that when we are studying a North Indian group and a South Indian group, educational differentials in child mortality are significantly smaller for the South Indian group.[9] We would like to hazard two (not mutually exclusive) explanations for this regional difference in the educational response:

1. Selectivity I.   In the Uttar Pradesh sample, where there is a smaller tradition of female literacy and education, the women who have had some schooling represent a special group for whom education is simply one more reflection of their households' greater receptivity to innovation. The selectivity argument is supported by the finding that in our Uttar Pradesh sample, among the educated women, 77 per cent have had four or more years of schooling while for Tamil Nadu, this figure is much lower at 54 per cent.[10]

2. Selectivity II.   According to this argument, Tamil Nadu as a whole represents a selective population, firstly because overall literacy levels are relatively very high (23 per cent in our sample, as opposed to 11 per cent in our Uttar Pradesh sample), so that there has been a trickle down or diffusion of ideas and household practices to the uneducated as well; secondly, and more importantly, the Tamil cultural background (which is associated with a whole range of characteristics such as greater maternal autonomy within and outside the household, greater female interaction with the outside world, greater and longer exposure to a modern medical care system) acts in the same way as education does in a more traditional culture. That is, the fact of being Tamil itself

Table 5.17. Infant and childhood mortality according to maternal education

	Uttar Pradesh			Tamil Nadu		
	Maternal education			Maternal education		
	None	Some	Some/none	None	Some	Some/none
% of children dead	26.8	15.9	0.6	24.7	18.2	0.8
% dying within[a]						
1 week	6.2	2.8	0.5	5.4	4.2	0.8
1 month	8.7	6.4	0.7	7.0	5.0	0.7
1–11 months	7.3	6.4	0.9	6.5	5.6	0.9
1–4 years	8.2	3.4	0.4	7.9	7.7	1.0

[a]These figures include only those live births that occurred before the relevant death interval and could have therefore been theoretically exposed to death in that interval.

means a greater willingness to try new kinds of behaviour, so that the effect of education is somewhat diluted.

This cultural base, to our minds, explains the lower educational differentials in child mortality and in the proximate determinants of child mortality in our South Indian sample. Even more significantly it explains why our uneducated South Indian mothers show better values for several of these proximate determinants than even the educated mothers from the Uttar Pradesh group. In fact, in the stages of origin (Registrar General of India 1981*a*), even infant mortality differentials by education show this pattern: the rural Infant Mortality Rate for uneducated women in Tamil Nadu in 1978 was 128, while for educated women in Uttar Pradesh it was 141 per 1000 live births. We will soon defend this conclusion empirically, but first there is the question of the educational impact on childhood deaths at different ages.

Table 5.17 suggests that while for Tamil Nadu the (relatively low) educational differential in mortality is more or less the same for all ages at death, in the case of Uttar Pradesh the no education/ some education ratio of 1.7 for all deaths hides some sharp differences in the effects of education at different ages: the effect is greatest at the perinatal stage (that is, immediately after birth) and in early childhood mortality (that is, in the 1–4 year age-group); post-neonatal mortality shows the smallest differentials by education of mother.

How does all this fit in with observed educational differences in the proximate determinants of child mortality? Very well, it appears from Table 5.18. The greatest educational differentials for Uttar Pradesh seem to be in those variables affecting neonatal and then early child mortality. The first two variables in the list—the percentage of births occurring in hospital and the percentage of mothers who begin breast-feeding a child on the day of birth—are important influences on neonatal mortality as already discussed in the earlier section. And both of them, especially the level of hospital deliveries, are strongly connected with maternal education. The third variable—the percentage of mothers who boil the water given to babies—is also strongly connected and is especially important in neonatal mortality in the present context where the initiation of breastmilk is delayed and some water-based substitute given.

Except for parity (row 4), none of the demographic variables usually implicated in infant and child mortality show a significant differential by education of mother. As discussed earlier in this chapter, fertility seems to affect childhood (that is 1–4 years) rather than infant mortality. Then, there are slight breast-feeding differentials by mother's education, but once again, given the usually long duration of breast-feeding in both educational groups, these differentials are not likely to be important predictors of mortality in infancy. And in the second year of life, when breast-feeding ends slightly earlier for the children of educated mothers, the potential dangers of this are compensated by the other illness preventive factors such as greater immunization and household hygiene.

Finally, we have the intermediate variables related to personal illness control. The most important education-related variable seems to be not the treatment of illness (which is in fact often more involved in the uneducated groups), but the level of prophylactic care. The educational differential in the percentage of children of Uttar Pradesh mothers who have received at least one dose of the triple antigen vaccination is large enough (see row 9, column 4); when it comes to the complete prescribed regimen of three doses of vaccine (row 10, column 4), the contrast between the educated and uneducated mothers is even sharper, with over three times as many children of educated mothers as those of uneducated mothers being allowed to take the full and therefore effective course of vaccinations.

How do the two regional groups compare in the extent of the maternal educational difference in the intermediate determinants of child mortality? In the same way as they do in their maternal educational differences in child mortality itself. To begin with, for each of the proximate determinants, the educational differential is much smaller for the Tamil Nadu sample than the Uttar Pradesh one. Secondly, there is obviously some other regional factor involved as well: the uneducated women from Tamil Nadu do better even than the educated women from Uttar Pradesh on several of these intermediate variables. For example, as many as 32 per cent of live births to the uneducated Tamil Nadu mothers have occurred in hospital, a figure which is of course way above the 6 per cent of births to uneducated Uttar Pradesh women that have had a similar type of delivery, but is also considerably larger than the figure of 15 per cent of births

Table 5.18. Maternal education and the proximate determinants of infant and childhood mortality

Nature of proximate determinant	Uttar Pradesh			Tamil Nadu		
	Maternal education			Maternal education		
	None	Some	Some/none	None	Some	Some/none
(1)	(2)	(3)	(4)	(5)	(6)	(7)
1. % of live births born in hospital	5.9	14.7	2.5	32.0	48.0	1.5
2. % of mothers who begin breastmilk within 1 day of birth	6.5	8.9	1.4	32.6	42.6	1.3
3. % of mothers who always boil the water fed to babies	16.9	45.2	2.7	27.4	50.4	1.8
4. Mean number of children ever born to women	4.1	2.2	0.5	3.6	3.0	0.8
5. Mean preceding interval for live births (months)	29.9	30.4	1.0	31.1	28.4	0.9
6. Mean succeeding interval for live births (months)	29.9	30.4	1.0	31.0	28.4	0.9
7. Mean maternal age at birth for live births (years)	23.4	23.2	1.0	23.0	22.2	1.0
8. Mean maternal duration of breast-feeding of living children	24.8	22.6	0.9	21.3	18.8	0.9

9. % of living children with at least one dose of triple antigen	33.6	59.1	1.8	39.7	36.1	0.9
10. % of living children with all 3 doses of triple antigen	7.2	22.7	3.2	25.7	21.9	0.9
11. % of illnesses in longitudinal study that received no treatment	15.4	13.3	0.9	16.1	19.0	1.2

to educated Uttar Pradesh mothers that have taken place in hospitals. The same remark applies to immunization, to the initiation of breastmilk on the day of birth, and to the boiling of water fed to babies. It should be mentioned that for both regional groups, education (at least in our kind of poor, slightly educated population) does not seem to really change ideas about disease causation and non-medical interventions. This point has also been made by, among others, Caldwell, Reddy, and Caldwell (1983) and Lindenbaum (1985). For example, there are no large educational differences in views on matters such as food intake during pregnancy or liquid intake during a bout of diarrhoea.

So much for maternal education. While the details vary, similar (though often less sharp) differences in child mortality and its proximate determinants are seen in our study for other socio-economic variables. The two consistent points which emerge are that differentials in the Tamil Nadu sample are usually smaller than in the Uttar Pradesh one and that within each socio-economic category, there are sharp regional differences in the values of the various mortality and proximate determinant variables, suggesting forcefully that it is not variations in socio-economic background which are mainly responsible for regional differentials in child mortality, and that cultural identity is an independent and powerful determinant of the intermediate variables and the various mortality outcomes which result.

Maternal Occupation

It is worth turning briefly now to maternal work status and child mortality, if only because even the broad results are not as predictable as in the maternal education case. Table 5.19 presents our data on the relationship between maternal work status and child mortality experience for the South Indian sample.[11] The contrast between the working and non-working groups is startling to say the least. Larger-scale data from the census, presented in Table 5.20, confirm this troubling finding. In each of the nine states, $q(5)$ is higher for working mothers.

At first sight this finding seems to contradict the wealth of our accumulated knowledge on the positive effects of women's economic independence. But that is not true. We do believe that economic power gives women precisely those freedoms and

Table 5.19. Maternal employment and childhood mortality:
field results for the Tamil Nadu sample

	Working mothers	Non-working mothers
q (2)	.1005	.0992
q (3)	.2330	.1472
q (5)	.2590	.1700
Average mortality level	13.93	16.97
Graduated q (2)	.1702	.1257
Graduated q (3)	.1892	.1372
Graduated q (5)	.2050	.1469

Note: q (x) values are based on the South family of life-tables and Trussell's equation. Graduated q (x) values are the q (x) values in the South model life table system corresponding to the average mortality level.

equalities that are associated with increased child survival when they arise from other sources, such as education or the absence of physical seclusion or even just the knowledge that employment is a socially acceptable option. It is just that in the case of actual employment there appears to be a crucial trade-off between

Table 5.20. Maternal employment and childhood mortality:
1981 census estimates

Region/State	q (5) for non-working women	q (5) for working women	$\frac{3-2}{2}$
(1)	(2)	(3)	(4)
All India	157	179	0.18
North			
Haryana	145	165	0.14
Madhya Pradesh	187	220	0.18
Punjab	122	131	0.07
Rajasthan	177	206	0.16
Uttar Pradesh	201	209	0.04
South			
Andhra Pradesh	128	162	0.27
Karnataka	134	172	0.28
Kerala	73	102	0.68
Tamil Nadu	97	163	0.68

Source: Registrar General of India (1988), *Census of India 1981: Child Mortality Estimates for India,* Government of India, New Delhi.

such autonomy and other factors detrimental to child survival. Of course, much fault can be found with the indicators used in Tables 5.19 and 5.20. In particular, are we actually looking at the effects of other kinds of socio-economic deprivation and bio-demographic variables rather than female employment *per se*? Detailed consideration of this possibility suggests that at least a part of the association is real (see United Nations 1985; Basu and Basu 1990). One needs therefore to search for possible routes through which poor populations suffer this one major disadvantage of women's employment.

To consider first the hypothesized ways in which working mothers can have a beneficial impact on child health and survival, the most important of these, of course, is the increased resources available for child welfare if the mother works. And as Mencher (1988) has graphically illustrated with data from villages in Tamil Nadu and Kerala, it is not just the fact of more money coming into the household that counts; what seems to matter is who brings in the extra money: with total household income remaining the same, a larger proportion of it seems to be spent on child welfare if the wife is working. Women's wages are more likely to be used for household (especially child) welfare than equivalent incomes earned by men. Similarly, Kumar (1977) concluded from fieldwork in Kerala that improvements in wage income were translated into improvements in child nutritional status more readily in households where the women were employed. With data from Panama, Tucker and Sanjur (1988) also concluded that maternal employment had a positive impact on children's dietary intakes. Popkin and Solon (1976) reached a similar conclusion in the Philippines, where mothers' work was found to have an independent effect on food expenditure.

The above kind of findings are consistent with the hypothesis that employment confers on women a greater command over resources and greater autonomy in decision-making, factors which have been attributed to education and held responsible for improved child survival by several writers, in particular Caldwell (see, for example, Caldwell 1986) in a series of papers on the relation between maternal education and child mortality. In our field study, for both regional groups, women who were employed took significantly greater responsibility for deciding on matters such as expenditure on food and clothing, what to cook, and how to treat an ill child. On the other hand, it must be added that working women often did worse on indicators such as watching television, going to the cinema, or talking to their husbands—we would attribute this not to greater seclusion but to a great shortage of time.

There is also likely to be a positive association between women's employment and access to knowledge about better childbearing and child-rearing practices, as well as a greater confidence and freedom in translating this knowledge into behaviour. This certainly seems to be the case where fertility-regulating behaviour is concerned, and there is no reason to believe that exposure to and willingness to accept health-related innovations are not similarly higher for working women. For instance, in the field study of the slum, working women were more likely to have had their deliveries take place in a hospital as opposed to the home (a possibly important influence on perinatal mortality; see Jain 1985) or to have initiated breast-feeding an infant within a day of birth.

One can think of other macro or community-level effects which would theoretically support a positive relationship between maternal employment and child survival as well. These effects operate through the negative two-way link between women's employment levels and their seclusion levels in a society, both in the literal and metaphorical sense. While the latter (that is, psychological seclusion) can affect child health through the kind of KAP (knowledge, attitude, and practice) variables mentioned above, the actual physical seclusion of women has important direct consequences for health. For example, in the urban study on which the primary data used here are based, the North Indian woman's greater reluctance to interact with the outside world was reflected in the very low proportions of hospital deliveries that occurred in this group (13 per cent as opposed to 32 per cent for the Tamil sample), even when the births took place in Delhi and therefore theoretically faced the same institutional choices as those facing the South Indians in the slum.

Even more invidious in their impact are health-affecting practices which have their roots in the restrictions on the physical movements of women and girls and which get more dangerous in the crowded and unhygienic environment of an urban slum. In our study, a large number of the women and girls from the Uttar

Pradesh households kept away from the public taps and toilets provided in the area: even among girls aged 10–12 years, as many as 51 per cent used the area just outside the home for urinating; 25 per cent even defecated there. The infection possibilites of such behaviour can well be imagined and it was no wonder that the North Indian lanes showed a higher incidence of gastro-intestinal ailments than the South Indian lanes in the slum.

What then is strong enough to override the above inventory of potential benefits of female employment status? One can think of several specific factors such as the ability to breast-feed (see in particularly the review chapters in Leslie and Paolisso 1989), but our evidence suggests that the more appropriate variable, though admittedly difficult to quantify, would be the quality and quantity of general child-care that the poor working mother can provide (the well-off working woman can, of course, make up for the quantity of her care with the quality of the substitute care available so that she experiences only the benefits of her work status).

Table 5.21 presents Indian survey data on child-care arrangements made by working mothers for 5-year-old girls in the rural areas (similar results obtain for boys and for the other ages). There seems to be a kind of North–South differential here as well, which is probably related to household structures as well as to differences in the occupational mix of working women in the different states. For example, a larger proportion of rural working women in the southern states work as labourers, while in the North they are more likely to be cultivators; the latter occupation is presumably more compatible with child-minding.

But even more interesting are percentages of children (at the age of 5!) who are reported to be looked after by no one when their mothers go to work (column 6 of Table 5.21). And now compare this with column 3 of Table 5.20 on the extent of the child mortality differential between working and non-working women in the different states. Except for Haryana, there seems to be a close association between this differential between working and non-working mothers and the proportion of children left to themselves. The southern states do the worst in this regard and the gap in child mortality between working and non-working mothers is the greatest for them. And Punjab and Uttar Pradesh seem to suffer the least, both in the extent of the child mortality

Table 5.21. Child-care when mother goes to
work: rural girls aged 5 years

State/region	Child's principal carer when mother at work (%)				
	Mother herself	Grand-parent	Other household member	Non-household member	No-one
(1)	(2)	(3)	(4)	(5)	(6)
All India	49	17	20	4	11
North					
Haryana	20	21	41	—	19
Madhya Pradesh	60	19	14	—	7
Punjab	43	44	14	—	—
Rajasthan	53	20	13	—	15
Uttar Pradesh	65	19	12	—	5
South					
Andhra Pradesh	43	16	27	7	8
Karnataka	46	12	16	7	20
Kerala	22	21	20	11	25
Tamil Nadu	43	6	18	10	24

Note: rules indicate numbers of negligible importance.

Source: Registrar General of India (1981), *Survey of Infant and Child Mortality 1979,* Government of India, New Delhi.

differential as well as in the proportion of children with no one to look after them.

Our hypothesis, therefore, is that a major explanation for the higher child mortality experience of working women can be found in their greater physical inability to look after their children themselves or to arrange adequate substitute child-care. This value of parental child-care is analogously suggested in studies which comment on the relationship between fertility and child mortality (see, for example, National Academy of Sciences 1989). It is also suggested in studies on the relation between maternal education and child mortality (for example, Caldwell 1986) which say that it is the mother who first notices a child's ill-health and the need to do something about it, and therefore if she is educated and free to act, the chances are greater that something will be done; whereas even if the father is educated and autonomous, his impact on child survival is smaller because he is less likely to be in a position to notice the ill-health in the first place. Restating this argument, even if the mother is autonomous and confident, she has to first be physically aware of a child's needs before she can move to meet them. Or perhaps it would be more correct to say that if one parent is employed or otherwise away, it is the other parent (not necessary biological), as opposed to other care-givers, whose attention most affects the detection and handling of ill-health in the child.

Besides care in ill-health, the general quality of child-care should also depend on the time available to the mother. For instance, Chaudhury's (1982) analysis of data from Bangladesh found that the time spent by the mother on child-care had a positive and significant effect on the calorie and protein intake and on the dietary adequacy status of pre-school children (see also Chutikul 1986).

Other studies on infant and child mortality which have looked in some detail at the primary care-giver reach similar conclusions. For example, Hilderbrand *et al.* (1985) have documented the significantly higher risks of death faced by children among the Tamasheq (or nobles) in rural Mali compared to the children of the Bella (or slaves). The latter can hardly claim to have greater economic resources; the main difference between the groups seems to be that Bella children are rarely physically separated from their mothers, whereas Tamasheq children are cared for by Bella nursemaids (who are often children themselves), being taken to their mothers only for breast-feeding. The authors stress the ignorance of Tamasheq mothers about their children's problems, the practice being to hand the child over to the servant at the slightest sign of troublesomeness. Similarly, Sussman (1980) has recorded the higher infant mortality of Parisian babies that were sent away to wet nurses in the country in the early nineteenth century, as compared to ordinary French infants. Even more revealing in the context of the present paper is the finding that the mortality of these children rose in the summer and autumn months; these were also the months in which agricultural employ-ment was more available to the wet nurses and made them perhaps less attentive to their charges.

If the relations discussed here are genuine (and we believe that they are), several policy implications suggest themselves. Of these the most salient would be the encouragement of a later age at entry into the labour-force. Presumably this would be associated with a relative crowding of births in the first years of childbearing so that the woman does not always have a young child to care for. This kind of behaviour seems to be appearing in the industrialized countries and if the physical consequences of smaller birth intervals can be got around, then one can see maternal employment as becoming unconnected with child survival. At the same time this would also help keep down the discrimination against girls because, as discussed in the next chapter, there are strong indications that the overall level of female employment in a community has an important bearing on the sex ratio of childhood mortality. Secondly, there should be a direct attack on the intermediate variables through which the maternal employment–child mortality relationship operates. These would include the provision of better child-care facilities and maternal work conditions, but how possible this is in a typical Third World country, where so much female labour is outside the organized sector, is a moot question. Finally, one cannot overemphasize the importance of greater economic resources for household survival. Our results suggest that at similar levels of household income, working women experience higher child loss than non-working women. They do not say anything about the child survival possibilities in households where women do not work, but do not have the increased income associated with their work either.

5.4. Discussion

To summarize the findings so far, the earlier sections have implicated the following intermediate variables in our observed regional differentials in infant and child mortality:

1. Demographic factors. While the usual demographic factors such as maternal age, birth order, and (especially) birth interval do show a relationship with childhood mortality in our study, they are not so clearly involved in explaining regional differentials. Only the variables of sex and parity seem capable of accepting any responsibiliy in this way. Both these variables seem to exert their greatest effect in early childhood (that is, in the 1–4 year age-group).

2. Sanitation and hygiene. This variable is important in explaining the lower level of illness incidence in our Tamil Nadu

Table 5.22. Regional differentials in childhood mortality:
Uttar Pradesh/Tamil Nadu ratio of deaths at different ages

Uttar Pradesh/Tamil Nadu ratios	Years since birth		
	5–9	15 +	All ages
All dead children	1.12	1.30	1.11
Children dying within			
1 week	1.41	1.13	1.15
1 month	1.39	1.23	1.26
1–11 months	1.08	1.72	1.17
1–5 years	0.91	1.38	1.01
1 year	1.21	1.42	1.22
5 years	1.11	1.40	1.18

Source: derived from Table 4.3.

children as compared to those from Uttar Pradesh households.
It should also be noted that the onset of breast-feeding represents
an important component of this intermediate variable.

3. Personal illness control. The two components of this proximate determinant which affect regional levels of child mortality
appear to be (*a*) antenatal care and institution of delivery, which
would be expected to influence perinatal and neonatal mortality
and (*b*) immunization, which would affect mortality via the
incidence of illness. Health care in illness does not seem to be
important at least in explaining regional differentials in recent
mortality, that is, mortality of children whose households are
theoretically exposed to the same health services.

These conclusions coincide surprisingly well with observed
regional differences in the age pattern of childhood mortality.
Table 5.22 looks at the Uttar Pradesh/Tamil Nadu ratio of the
percentages of children dying in different age intervals for two
groups of children—one relatively young and the other older—as
well as for all children together.

To begin with the younger children, Table 5.22 shows clearly
that the largest regional differential occurs in perinatal and
neonatal morality. This is the stage of life when the mortality
determinants are primarily biological and those related to the
conditions of birth. Biologically, we have no reason to believe that
the Tamil household has any great advantages. But where birth
conditions are concerned, the regional differences are clear. Not

only do a much larger proportion of the Tamil women have their deliveries in a professional institution, but more importantly, they are also much more likely to have received some antenatal care during pregnancy. Moreover, and as importantly, a much larger proportion of the Tamil women begin breast-feeding their babies soon after birth, therefore not just providing the nutrition and antibodies essential in early life but also preventing the infections caused by breastmilk substitutes which are generally dissolved in unboiled water.

There is a sharp fall in the regional differential in mortality once we reach the post-neonatal and early childhood stages. We believe that modern medical care is the great equalizer here. As our data have consistently demonstrated, there are no real differences in the unalloyed faith in modern doctors between the two groups, once services are controlled. If anything, the Uttar Pradesh household's belief in its miraculous properties is greater and this is possibly what explains the regional ratio of mortality in the 1–4 year age-group being below unity. In fact this impact of health care is strong enough to overcome the North Indian sample's disadvantages in preventive health care—both household hygiene and immunization of children. However, we did mention that the one regional difference in the handling of illness by the two groups was the much greater resort to self-treatment at home for illnesses in infants from Uttar Pradesh. Consistent with this, the regional ratio for mortality in the 1–11 months age-group is significantly higher than it is for deaths between the ages of one and four years in Table 5.22.

For older cohorts of children on the other hand, the regional ratio is the highest for post-neonatal and childhood mortality; not surprisingly, since these children represent a cohort of unequal access to health care, or at least their mothers represent a cohort with unequal experience of the modern health-care system. In such a situation not only are the children from Uttar Pradesh at a relatively greater disadvantage because their illnesses have a greater chance of being fatal, they also suffer because their morbidity levels are higher as a result of more inadequate household hygiene and immunization levels.

How does the status of women relate to the above pattern of regional differences in child mortality? This question is best answered by seeking a connection (however qualitative) between the status of women and those proximate determinants implicated in the regional child mortality differential:

1. Sex. The link between women's status and sex differences in mortality is discussed more fully in the next chapter. Here, it will suffice to say that women's roles as defined by their cultural background influence gender differences in physical well-being through both positive discrimination in favour of boys as well as inadvertent discrimination due to the customs and fears bred by the norms of female seclusion and economic dependence.

2. Parity. The previous chapter has already discussed the ways in which women's position is linked to regional differences in fertility behaviour. To recapitulate, once more there are two pathways of influence, the level of son preference, and the knowledge of, attitude towards, and practice of birth-control independent of family size desires.

3. Sanitation and hygiene. Differences in women's levels of seclusion and in their ability to interact freely with the outside world were hypothesized in this chapter to lead to differences in their levels of knowledge about behaviour conducive to health as well as in their ability to act on this knowledge even when it was acquired. For example, the urban slum environment was found to be particularly well suited to the spread of gastro-intestinal infections because of the insecurity felt by the North Indians about sending young girls to public toilets.

4. Nutrition. While there were many differences in the nutritional behaviour of the two groups, women's position was found to be important in two specific ways. In the North Indians, the lack of information and lower autonomy in decision-making led to one major nutritional practice being worse in this group: the practice of delaying the onset of breast-feeding until about the third day after birth. In the case of the South Indians, their increased interaction with the outside world led to two potentially deleterious health practices: shorter durations of breast-feeding, and relatively infrequent cooking of food in a situation of poor food preservation and storage facilities. However, on balance, at least on the child survival score, the Tamil women's adverse practices probably had less of an impact than those of their northern counterparts.

5. Health-care use. In this, the Uttar Pradesh women were found to be disadvantaged in two specific ways: firstly, in their

relatively poor use of antenatal care and, relatedly, relatively poor use of modern health facilities for childbirth; and secondly, in their poorer compliance with the rules for effective immunization. Of these, the former, together with the delayed onset of breast-feeding mentioned above, undoubtedly accounted for at least a part of the regional difference in perinatal mortality, while the latter worked through its effect on illness incidence. And both these factors were also postulated to be due to the fears and poor access to information that resulted from the women's seclusion and economic dependence.

Surprisingly, in the aggregate figures, curative health-care use was not found to be affected by regional factors. However, as the next chapter elucidates, these aggregate figures hide important age and sex differentials in the use of health-care services. The sex differential was particularly important because a reduction in the sex imbalance in child mortality would also considerably narrow the regional difference in overall mortality.

The role of women's status indicators was also suggested by the lower impact of factors such as maternal education on child mortality and it proximate determinants among the South Indians. This was consistent with the lower impact of education on more direct measures of women's status described in Chapter 3. Moreover, a partial cultural explanation for the regional differential in child mortality was further supported by the finding that even when one looked only at uneducated women, the Tamils experienced better child survival than the women from Uttar Pradesh. Indeed, if one could discount the negative impact of their work on child survival, the regional difference would be even greater: compare child mortality levels for all (that is, primarily non-working) North Indian women in Table 5.1 with those for non-working Tamil women in Table 5.19. At the same time, the women's position variables continue to overcome several of the disadvantages of employment among the South Indians; even working South Indian women, who do so much worse than their non-working South Indian counterparts, still manage to experience better child survival than the North Indian women: once more, compare Tables 5.1 and 5.19.

We are now in a position to complete the right-hand side of the women's status–demographic behaviour model for the variable child mortality, as shown in Fig. 5.1. This figure is not really as

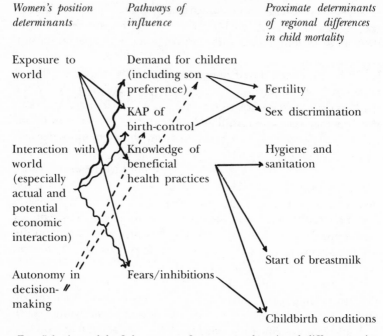

Fig. 5.1. A model of the status of women and regional differences in child mortality

much of a jungle as it looks. To put it more generally, other socio-economic factors being constant,

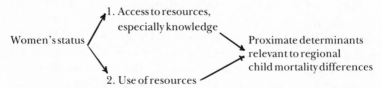

Finally, we turn to Table 5.23. We believe that there is something called the household level of mortality. That is, some households have a greater propensity to child deaths than others. This is seen in the sharp rise in the percentages of children dead once we move from children with no dead sibling to children with one or more dead siblings. To expand on this, the probability that a household with two dead children will experience a third child loss is significantly greater than the probability that a household with one dead child will experience a second child loss.

Table 5.23. % children dead according to number of dead siblings

Number of dead siblings	Uttar Pradesh (N=2420)			Tamil Nadu (N=1937)		
	Number of siblings ever born					
	1–2	3–5	6 +	1–2	3–5	6 +
0	15.4	16.4	27.6	11.1	18.0	37.5
1	19.6	22.3	39.0	20.4	28.5	30.6
2 +	56.3	24.9	45.9	0.0	26.8	40.3

This is reasonable if one accepts that, quite apart from child mortality which is selective in some way (for example by sex or birth order), households also have a base of ingrained patterns of health-related behaviour (for example, hygienic practices, faith in vaccinations) which operate across all children and which are also slow to change. Such an interpretation probably also partly explains Hobcraft, McDonald, and Rutstein's (1985) finding that the adverse effects on child mortality of the preceding birth interval are even greater if the previous child dies than when it survives.

We close this chapter by emphasizing again the central theme of this study: that whatever the proximate determinants that influence child survial, regional differentials in these proximate determinants persist after controlling for the usual socio-economic characteristics such as education, occupation, and caste. That is, the cultural background, especially as it affects the position of women, itself contributes in a significant way to the observed differentials in the intermediate variables of mortality and in mortality itself.

NOTES

1. In particular, see Palloni (1989) for an illuminating discussion on the difficulties involved in correctly understanding and interpreting the strong and apparently universal relationship between birth intervals and child mortality.
2. At the same time, prematurity may not be a confounding variable to the extent that it is encouraged by closely spaced pregnancies.
3. We make no mention here of the prohibitive cost of fuel to our households. Indeed, taking this into account, these attempts to

promote infant health are admirable. But the concern here is with the regional differential which exists in spite of the absence of an economic differential by region of origin.

4. This is a universal problem, as seen, for example, in the conclusion by Oddy (1970) on examining nineteenth-century English diets that the average low-income Englishman could have had a much more nutritious diet at a lower price if he had been prepared to change his consumption patterns. This might be a contributory factor in the observed paradox between the rise in real wages and the low standards of nutrition and health in England at the turn of the twentieth century.

5. The high level of non-vegetarianism in the Tamil sample is because of the over-representation of the lower castes. In the higher castes, vegetarianism is wellnigh universal even today.

6. But, conversely to the Uttar Pradesh sample, this is still a reduction in the percentages from those occurring in hospital in Tamil Nadu itself. This is probably a result of the greater ignorance and insecurity of the Tamil women after moving to the capital city, especially as they face a major language problem when they first arrive.

7. Or so one believed, until the well-publicized curious case of the baby that changed its sex in one of the large public hospitals in the city: a woman who had delivered a male child according to the hospital records and the testimony of her own eyes, was suddenly given a female infant to feed about a week after the delivery. The male baby seemed to have disappeared completely and the wild theories that were floated to explain the disappearance were a fitting reflection of the 'son mania' that exists in this area.

8. However, it is quite likely that accessibility itself is influenced by cultural factors, with some groups being more demanding in their desire for modern health services. This is believed to be the case, for example, in Kerala (see Nag 1983), and even in our study the Tamil group felt much more strongly that one of the main facilities which were inadequate in their area was that for health. In fact we were urged on several occasions to use our imagined influence to do something about this.

9. Micro-level evidence from different parts of the country confirms this finding that the maternal education impact on child survival is larger in the northern part of the country. For example, Khan (1988) found a very strong relationship between mother's education and infant mortality in rural Uttar Pradesh. In contrast, both Gunasekaran (1988) and Ramanujam (1988) reported from their field data from Tamil Nadu that there were no significant differentials in infant mortality according to the literacy status of the mother.

10. This may also partly explain why the educated women from Uttar

Pradesh have experienced smaller child loss than the educated women from Tamil Nadu.

11. The Uttar Pradesh sample had too few working women to make a meaningful comparison. But, even with this constraint, the general result was the same as for the South Indians in the study.

6

Sex Differences
in Physical Well-Being

UNTIL recently, most research in the social sciences was content to stop at the household as the unit of analysis. It was assumed that the interests, views, and welfare of the different individuals who constituted a household were identical and that broader classifications such as class and caste reflected more important and relevant distinctions. However, in recent years, the appropriateness of this view has been increasingly questioned in a spate of studies and, especially with the rise of a feminist consciousness, we seem about to swing completely the other way, denying the existence of any kind of common family or household interests. While such a complete swing would again be self-defeating, this new focus on household members as separate individuals has served an essential purpose in identifying more sharply the high-risk groups in a population (that is, those most urgently in need of attention); this being a particularly useful purpose in situations where the resources available for improvements in welfare are limited.

This chapter tries to explore intra-household differentials in the theoretically least controversial area of welfare, the physical quality of life, and to relate these to women's status as an important determining variable. It steers clear of more abstract issues such as intra-household differences in happiness, rights, and the fulfillment of desires, an area which has begun to generate a substantial literature in philosophy in the last few years. As can be imagined, the conceptual and measurement problems involved in this enterprise are immense. Nor does this chapter touch upon subjective matters such as people's perceptions about their level of physical welfare. Given the conditioning and incomplete access to information that characterize (especially a traditional) society, what people believe about even a relatively straightforward matter such as their health problems need not have any connection with what the doctor believes. In this light, the finding from the Singur study in West Bengal (see Kynch and Sen 1983) that about half the widowers interviewed after the Bengal famine of 1943 complained that they were in indifferent health, compared to a mere 2.5 per cent of the widows, is interesting, but not because it is unexpected.

I also leave out a discussion on intra-household differences in more tangible factors such as access to and use of education and employment opportunities, which do, of course, have an indirect connection with physical welfare. It hardly needs stressing that there are important inequalities even within a household in the distribution of these resources, especially in some parts of the region. It is also one of the ground rules of this chapter that greater equality in this distribution is essential for removing internal disparities in ultimate physical welfare.

But for the present I concentrate on intra-family differences in the immediate physical quality of life. I use three indicators of the quality of life: mortality, nutritional status, and health status. While the focus here is on differences in these indicators according to sex, one should perhaps also add that age is a prominent variable in determining intra-household differences. But age is given secondary importance here, first, because differentials by age tend to be less severe than those by sex, and secondly, because they are less invidious in a sense since age, unlike gender, is not fixed and (at least in principle) all individuals stand some chance of passing through the more favourable ages at some time. Moreover, age differentials in welfare are considered briefly in the previous chapter.

While this chapter relies on primary data for the bulk of the discussion and especially for delineating the finer details of arguments, more use is made of secondary sources here than in the rest of this book. This is because increasingly sophisticated large-scale secondary data are becoming available to draw a broader picture to complement the results of micro-studies such as ours, and because wherever possible a consideration of secular trends is an important aid to understanding contemporary levels and differentials.

While I venture briefly into the subject of gender differences at older ages, the focus is on the very young; that is, children up to the age of five. Besides the fact that our data are most complete for this age-group, such a focus is warranted because gender differences in physical welfare seem to be the most pronounced among young children. And even when they are not, the experience of young children, especially in the case of mortality, provides a large proportion of the experience of the population as a whole. This is especially so for South Asia, where child mortality relative to adult mortality seems to be much higher for any given mortality level, compared to standard models of mortality based on non-South Asian populations.

While the overall framework of this chapter is one for understanding discrimination as it affects the ultimate outcome of physical well-being, mortality, gender differences in nutrition and in health are considered in independent sections and not merely as correlates of mortality because, even when they do not result in mortality, they are very meaningful indicators of the general quality of life for individuals, as well as of the general air of discrimination within the household.

Wherever the evidence does point to important sex differences in the physical quality of life, an attempt is made in this chapter to relate these to both socio-economic and cultural variables, especially those believed to be associated with the status of women as outlined in Chapter 3. In practice this means that the effect of women's status on sex differences in child mortality, exposure to illness, and health care in illness is considered in some detail. Other indicators of physical well-being, such as nutritional status and prophylactic medical care, turn out not to exhibit significant or consistent gender differentials. There is a continued focus on regional variations in sex differences in these aspects of physical welfare, given the primary hypothesis of this book that regional differentials in the position of women are associated with regional differentials in demographic behaviour, including sex differences in survival.

6.1. Mortality

It is by now clear that the sex pattern of mortality in several parts of South Asia and some parts of the Middle East is quite different from that in the rest of the world, with females exhibiting higher rates of mortality than males, especially in childhood and the reproductive span. This difference is seen whatever the kind of evidence one examines: population sex ratios from censuses (for example, Visaria 1967; El-Badry 1969); the more appropriate juvenile sex ratios which control to some extent for sex-selective migration (for example, Sopher 1980; Miller 1981) and more recently, even direct estimates of death-rates (for example, Registrar General of India 1981*a*; D'Souza and Chen 1980; Langford 1984; Das Gupta 1987).

We begin this section with a brief discussion on trends in the sex ratio of mortality in India. Table 6.1 presents trends in the sex ratio of the enumerated population in successive Indian censuses, the simplest measure of possible sex differentials in mortality in largely closed populations. This sex ratio appears to be consistently in favour of males. Superficially, it suggests that up to 1971 at least, the female disadvantage in survival has continuously increased. However, as Dyson (1988) points out, this is not strictly true. Up to about 1921 there is a female advantage in survival, given a sex ratio at birth of 104 to 106 males per 100 females and the sex ratio of the population never exceeding this figure. Indeed, in the 1901 census there is an actual decrease in the masculinity of the population because males seem to have suffered

Table 6.1. Trends in the sex ratio of the
Indian population, 1881–1991

Census year	Population sex ratio (males per 1000 females)
1881	1039
1891	1039
1901	1029
1911	1038
1921	1047
1931	1053
1941	1058
1951	1057
1961	1063
1971	1075
1981	1069
1991	1076

Source: Registrar General of India (1991), *Census of India 1991: Provisional Population Totals*, Government of India, New Delhi.

disproportionately more in the famines of 1897 and 1900. In fact it is only around 1941, as mortality came more within control, that the real disadvantage to females begins. At the same time, the picture for females is worse than it appears from these aggregate figures because there has continued to be an excess of males in the population in spite of the biological advantage that females have in neonatal as well as old-age mortality: an advantage that is enough to bring down the sex ratio of the population to below unity in several other parts of the world. These figures cannot simply be attributed to underdevelopment. For example, if the Indian sex ratio in the 1981 population had been similar to that of another undeveloped region such as Africa, India would have had 30 million more women; Sen (1987) has called these the 'missing women' in India's demography.

The second period during which females seem to regain some lost ground is during 1971–81. But, once again, it is not clear how much of the decline in the sex ratio is due to a narrowing of sex differentials in mortality and how much due to a greater under-enumeration of women during the 1971 census; probably both factors are relevant. But we can speculate with greater knowledge on the possibilities during this period because of several sources of data on death-rates. I now look at some of these to understand intra-household differences in the risks of death.

To concentrate on deaths in early childhood, that is by the age of 5, Table 6.2 presents indirect estimates of the probability of dying by this age, from the 1981 census. The table suggests that by this time, the sharp female disadvantage in survival was no longer the rule in all parts of the country and confirms Dyson's (1989) conclusion from a series of independent data sources that the country as a whole seemed to have almost 'crossed over' from a position of higher child mortality for girls to one where boys did worse on this score.

However, it is worth noting that the first provisional results of the 1991 census (Registrar General of India, 1991) suggest a return to the old trend; once more, there is a rise in the masculinity of the population. It is too early to attribute this rise with any confidence to specific factors, and it may well be that the last three decades (that is, the period of greatest mortality decline) have seen no trend, only fluctuations around a mean population sex ratio of around 1070 males per 1000 females. But a rise in the population

Table 6.2. Regional differentials in the sex ratio of
childhood mortality

State	q(5)		q(5) Boys ÷ q(5) Girls	Sex ratio (males per 100 females) of children ever born to women aged 30–34
	Boys	Girls		
All India	.147	.157	.94	105
Andhra Pradesh	.143	.135	1.06	102
Bihar	.131	.153	.86	110
Gujarat	.085	.090	.94	108
Haryana	.123	.153	.82	114
Karnataka	.143	.140	1.02	105
Kerala	.085	.076	1.12	105
Madhya Pradesh	.193	.201	.96	109
Maharashtra	.146	.144	1.01	107
Orissa	.123	.122	1.01	NA
Punjab	.104	.118	.88	114
Rajasthan	.166	.186	.89	111
Tamil Nadu	.134	.131	1.02	105
Uttar Pradesh	.174	.208	.84	113
West Bengal	.073	.074	.99	107

Source: Registrar General of India (1988), *Census of India 1981. Child Mortality Estimates of India,* Government of India, New Delhi; Registrar General of India (1981); and (for each state), *Census of India 1981, Report and Tables Based on 5% Sample Data,* Government of India, New Delhi.

sex ratio during a decade of further falls in mortality and with little reason to expect the selective under-enumeration of females to have increased, does suggest that a widening of the gap between male and female mortality is not implausible.

For one thing, if the fall in overall mortality has been largely a function of better health services (as seems to be the case), and given the weight of the evidence on sex differentials in access to and use of health care, discussed later in this chapter, it would not be surprising if the mortality decline had accrued disproportionately to males. Secondly, there may have been a rise in the sex differential in mortality if different causes of death exhibited different rates of decline over time. For instance, one may speculate that a major fall in young adult mortality from respiratory diseases would positively affect the survival chances of males more that females, as the former seem to succumb more readily to these.

The other pathway to changes in population sex ratios involves no change in the sex ratio of mortality within various socio-economic groups, but changes in the distribution of such groups. For example, census data as well as data from smaller studies in India and abroad suggest that educated women, while they experience lower absolute levels of childhood mortality, may simultaneously experience greater gender differences in such mortality compared to their uneducated counterparts. And, given the rises in female education and literacy over the last decade, the experience of educated women may now account for a larger proportion of total mortality experience than in the 1981 census.

Similarly, the impact of female employment may be important. As discussed later in this chapter, it seems to be the case that the children of working women tend to face more equal survival chances by sex than those of non-working women. As yet, we have no readily comparable data on trends in female employment, but if these are negative, they could well result in an overall increase in the sex differential in mortality. One indication of the possibility of declines in female employment at the lower socio-economic levels is the traditional U-shaped relationship between female education and employment. We may now be at the base of this U, with medium levels of female education and hence the lowest levels of female employment on the curve.

Moreover, the sex ratio of the population has also not been able to reap one potential benefit. If the decline in fertility had been more substantial, perhaps the overall sex differential in mortality would have been reduced; this differential is greater for higher order births.

On the whole, therefore, it appears that a small but significant increase in the sex differential in mortality could have taken place at the national level and may account for at least a part of the increase in the population sex ratio. Age breakdowns of the population will allow a better assessment of this possibility. Incidentally, it is probably increasingly important to take into account possible changes in the sex ratio of births as one factor in the rising population sex ratio. Premi (1991) has speculated that this may be occurring with better health conditions and consequent falls in intra-uterine mortality (which are biased against male foetuses).

In addition, recent years have also seen the unanticipated interference of a technological advance which may soon exert an impact on the population sex ratio. The increasingly easy availability of the amniocentesis procedure to detect the sex of the foetus, as well as the Medical Termination of Pregnancy procedure for legalized abortions, have resulted, in some localized areas at least, in a rush to abort female foetuses and, consequently, a possibly artificial rise in the sex ratio of births.

At a wider state or national level, it is difficult to conclude anything definite about the role of such artificially induced changes in the sex ratio of births in influencing changes in the sex ratio of the population. While indications are that sex determination tests are becoming more and more socially acceptable, we may be exaggerating their current extent at a national level, especially since medical evidence suggests that as yet the amniocentesis procedure cannot reliably predict the sex of the foetus in the first weeks of a pregnancy; so a significant proportion of the abortions that follow the test may actually be male. Moreover, even if they were predominantly female, it is not clear that all these aborted foetuses would otherwise have been born or would have survived until the census.

In any case, I would include the effects of sex-selective abortions in the category of sex differentials in mortality because that is what they amount to; the only difference is in the age at death, which now needs to include a 'minus 5–8 months' category.

Moreover, it is important to point out that even in 1981, and perhaps at present as well, there are significant regional differentials in the sex ratio of childhood mortality. As Table 6.2 brings out, on the whole it appears that the northern and north-western parts of the country continue to be plagued by higher female mortality in early childhood, while in the South, the greater biological hardiness of the female has begun to assert itself. In addition, one needs to make two corrections which suggest that the male–female imbalance in the risk of death from exogenously determined causes is probably higher than that shown in Table 6.2.

1. For all states, neonatal mortality (that is, deaths in the first month of life) is included in the $q(5)$ estimates. However, neonatal

mortality (of which endogenous causes are a heavy component) is significantly higher for boys and therefore the exogenously determined female disadvantage of girls is greater than an all-inclusive figure of child mortality suggests.

2. The last column of Table 6.2 implies under-reporting of dead girls in the northern states; this is why we get a sex ratio of live births of over 110 males per 100 females instead of (a more likely) 104–106. This again means that female mortality is under-estimated and, therefore, so is the sex differential in mortality. But one should perhaps mention Dyson's (1989) contention that at least a part of the high reported sex ratio of births in North India may be caused by a tendency for women to under-report daughters living away from home. But this bias is likely to be greater, among the older women, who are more likely to have married daughters. Such an interpretation is particularly appealing for North Indian women, for whom village exogamy means a greater physical distance from married daughters, as discussed in Chapter 3. These two corrections lead one to the conclusion that we have not progressed as much as we could have in ensuring equal life chances for male and female births and that the regional contrast is even sharper than it appears in Table 6.2.

Once we leave the childhood ages behind, it appears that, after the peak childbearing years, male death-rates currently exceed female death-rates sufficiently for overall life expectancy at age 5 to have become higher for females since the late 1970s, even in rural areas. And at younger ages after the age of 5 but before the reproductive span of 20–34, girls are also fast losing their dis-advantage in survival. The reasons for the higher mortality of males at older ages are not clear. It has been suggested (see Dyson 1984) that respiratory illnesses, especially tuberculosis, may be the main culprit, being greater in incidence and severity in males because of various behavioural factors. Indeed in India, for both sexes, mortality in early childhood and in late adulthood is significantly higher than it was in Western populations when they were at a similar level of overall life expectancy. These intra-household differences in the age pattern of death probabilities need to be understood much better.

It is also worth pointing out that direct measures of mortality are essential to understand the situation at sub-national levels, where migration may be an important determinant of population sex ratios. In such cases, sex ratios favourable to women do not necessarily imply conditions of life favourable to women; if they are the result of male out-migration, they may actually imply a greater strain on women, who now live in what are effectively female-headed households, with all their attendant disadvantages in an economy that is labour-intensive and a society that is patriarchal.

Findings from the Primary Data

In the present survey too, although the two regional groups being studied have similar socio-economic levels and an identical external physical environment, their experience of childhood mortality showed the same kind of differences found in secondary data from the two states of origin. The Tamil women had both lower levels of proportions of children dead as well as smaller sex differences in the proportions of children dead as seen in Table 6.3. Indeed there is some reason to believe that the differences between the two cultural groups may be even more marked. Column 5 of Table 6.3 indicates an abnormally high sex ratio of births for Uttar Pradesh and in spite of our repeated probes to the women in this sample, it appears likely that there has been significant under-reporting of dead daughters. Assuming a more likely sex ratio of live births of even a relatively high figure such as 1.08 rather than the reported 1.14, raises the proportion of daughters dead from 0.27 to 0.31; which means that the sex ratio of child mortality (male–female) falls further from 0.86 to 0.76. For the Tamil sample, this corresponding sex ratio of live births is 1.03.

At this point, it is perhaps worth adding in our defence that the tendency to under-report dead daughters in our Uttar Pradesh sample is less a reflection of insufficient interviewer doggedness and more a cultural characteristic of the respondents themselves: even the 1981 census reported a sex ratio of 1.15 males per female for children ever born to women aged 15–49 in Uttar Pradesh, in both rural and urban areas (Registrar General of India 1983*a*). And in Tamil Nadu, this figure was closer to the expected, being 1.07.

In Table 6.4, the data from Table 6.3 have been converted to life-table parameters using Trussell's South model coefficients as described in the United Nations *Manual X* (1983). The South

Table 6.3. Regional differentials in sex ratios of children ever born and in proportions dead by sex

Region and age group of mothers	Mean number of children ever born	Proportion of sons dead	Proportion of daughters dead	Sex ratio (sons/daughters) of children ever born
Uttar Pradesh (N=618)				
15–19	0.68	.229	.063	1.09
20–24	2.23	.175	.262	1.17
25–29	3.69	.189	.226	1.20
30–34	4.34	.228	.258	1.07
35–39	4.57	.217	.289	1.20
40–44	5.48	.343	.305	1.12
45–49	5.96	.347	.389	1.01
All ages	3.76	.235	.273	1.14
Tamil Nadu (N=522)				
15–19	1.10	.520	.273	1.50
20–24	1.92	.175	.104	1.01
25–29	3.30	.179	.216	0.97
30–34	3.67	.211	.208	1.02
35–39	4.32	.254	.224	0.97
40–44	4.94	.246	.190	1.04
45–59	5.03	.261	.299	1.03
All ages	3.26	.212	.205	1.03

Table 6.4. Regional and sex differences in childhood mortality using the South family of model life-tables and Trussell's equation

Mortality indicator	Uttar Pradesh		Tamil Nadu	
	Boys	Girls	Boys	Girls
q(2)	.160	.241	.115	.081
q(3)	.183	.218	.182	.214
q(5)	.228	.259	.235	.220
Average mortality level	14.26	10.84	15.21	15.0
Graduated q(2)[a]	.172	.214	.157	.147
Graduated q(3)[a]	.190	.242	.173	.164
Graduated q(5)[a]	.205	.265	.186	.177

[a] Graduated q(x) values are the q(x) values in the South model life-table system corresponding to the average mortality level.

model of the Coale–Demeny set of model life-tables has been employed because it is the closest to the Indian situation of high mortality below age 5 relative to mortality above 5. It can be seen that girls from Uttar Pradesh have a much lower probability of surviving early childhood than boys, while in the case of Tamil Nadu, the two sexes face about equal chances; if anything, the female confirms her physical superiority over the male.

The initial survey of ever-married women was followed by a six-month longitudinal study which covered all children who were below the age of twelve and had at least one living sibling below twelve as well. Surprisingly (given the relatively small sample size and relatively short duration of the longitudinal study) the above regional and sex pattern of child deaths was repeated, as demonstrated in Table 6.5. The Uttar Pradesh sample showed a staggeringly low figure of 0.121 for the sex ratio (male–female) of child death-rates, while for Tamil Nadu this index reached unity.

Table 6.6 presents direct estimates of childhood mortality derived from the survival status of each individual live birth. The picture remains unchanged—for the Tamil sample we have 99 daughters dying for every 100 dead sons and for Uttar Pradesh 115—indeed, as our sex ratios of live births in Table 6.3 suggest, this second figure is likely to be an under-estimate. Table 6.6 has another interesting feature. This is the large number of female births to the Uttar Pradesh women for whom all that we know is that they were born and they died. When they were born is not

Table 6.5. Sex differentials in mortality among children under 12 during the six-month longitudinal study

| | Uttar Pradesh | | | | Tamil Nadu | | | |
| | Age-group | | | | Age-group | | | |
	< 5	5–9	10–12	All ages	< 5	5–9	10–12	All ages
Boys								
No. of deaths	2	0	0	2	2	1	0	3
Deaths/1000/year	15.0	0.0	0.0	7.0	32.8	19.1	0.0	23.3
No. in sample	267	209	94	570	122	105	31	258
Girls								
No. of deaths	9	3	2	14	3	0	0	3
Deaths/1000/year	78.3	34.5	49.4	57.7	49.2	0.0	0.0	22.7
No. in sample	230	174	81	485	122	106	37	265

Table 6.6. Sex differentials in childhood mortality: direct estimates

| | Years since birth | | | | | | | | | | | | | | |
| | <1 | | 1–4 | | 5–9 | | 10–14 | | 15+ | | N.S.[a] | | All ages | | All ages |
	M	F	M	F	M	F	M	F	M	F	M	F	M	F	M/F
A. Uttar Pradesh (N=2482)															
% children dead	8.8	5.6	12.1	16.2	20.9	26.8	25.3	27.5	37.5	39.7	85.7	100.0	24.5	28.5	0.86
% dying within:															
1 week			4.7	3.2	5.9	5.8	6.2	5.8	9.0	6.9	—	—	6.7	5.5	1.22
1 month			6.3	5.7	7.2	8.6	9.0	7.5	13.3	8.9	—	—	9.3	7.9	1.18
1–11 months			2.3	4.5	7.2	8.6	6.2	7.5	9.8	9.8	—	—	6.7	8.0	0.84
1–4 years			8.6	10.1	4.7	5.8	7.3	7.5	8.5	13.8	—	—	6.9	9.3	0.72
1 year					14.4	17.2	15.2	15.0	23.1	18.7	—	—	16.0	15.9	1.01
5 years					19.1	23.0	22.5	22.5	31.6	32.5	—	—	24.8	26.9	0.92
5–9 years							1.0	0.4	0.5	1.3	—	—	0.7	0.9	0.78
age at death not stated			0.8	3.6	1.6	3.8	1.0	3.3	4.3	3.3	—	—	2.5	4.2	0.59
B. Tamil Nadu (N=2007)															
% children dead	2.3	5.6	17.3	10.3	20.2	22.3	24.9	24.9	29.1	30.3	100.0	100.0	23.8	23.5	1.01
% dying within:															
1 week			4.5	4.0	5.6	2.8	5.1	1.7	8.9	5.6	—	—	6.6	4.0	1.65
1 month			5.6	5.2	7.5	3.8	5.7	2.9	10.9	7.6	—	—	8.1	5.4	1.50
1–11 months			6.7	2.9	4.7	10.0	8.5	8.1	5.1	6.3	—	—	5.9	6.8	0.87
1–4 years			12.3	8.1	6.6	4.7	9.6	11.0	6.1	10.1	—	—	7.0	8.7	0.81
1 year					12.2	13.8	14.2	11.0	16.0	13.9	—	—	14.0	12.3	1.14
5 years					18.8	18.5	23.8	22.0	22.1	24.0	—	—	21.4	22.0	0.97
5–9 years							0.6	1.2	1.0	1.0	—	—	0.9	1.1	0.82
Age at death not stated			1.1	0.5	1.4	2.4	0.6	1.1	2.0	2.5	—	—	2.0	2.1	0.95

Note: each of the rows includes only those births that occurred before the relevant age at death interval and could have therefore been theoretically exposed to death in that age interval.

[a] time of birth not stated..

stated and in a high proportion of these briefly mentioned births, the particulars of their death—age at death, cause of death, etc.—are not mentioned either. It is not clear if such forgetfulness is a genuine outcome of the lesser importance given to a female birth and its survival or a desire to hush up an event which stirs up uncomfortable feelings. But it is somewhat revealing that the educated women in our study, who presumably are able to keep a better record of their own maternity history (especially since this record is shorter, their fertility being lower), report a sex ratio of children ever born of 1.25, which is considerably higher than the mean sex ratio of 1.15 reported by their uneducated sisters (see also Ware 1984).

Socio-economic Influences on Sex Differences in Childhood Mortality

Counter to initial expectations, Table 6.7 suggests that the sex differential in child mortality rises with a rise in socio-economic factors such as income or caste. This finding brings us back to the central conclusion of this report: that the position of women is an integral variable in any attempt to understand demographic behaviour in the Third World. The increased sex differential in mortality with rises in socio-economic status, even though resources also presumably rise with such improvement in household status, fits in well with the frequently noted inverse

Table 6.7. Sex ratio of childhood mortality according to various socio-economic indicators

Socio-economic indicator	Uttar Pradesh (N=2482) % dead			Tamil Nadu (N=2007) % dead		
	Boys	Girls	Boys/girls	Boys	Girls	Boys/girls
Caste						
Lower	23.6	27.3	0.86	25.1	23.4	1.07
Upper	25.6	38.5	0.67	19.6	21.1	0.93
Mother's education						
None	25.3	28.4	0.89	24.3	25.2	0.96
Some	10.3	22.9	0.45	20.2	16.3	1.24
Mother's employment						
None	23.7	27.9	0.85	19.4	23.0	0.84
Some	32.6	30.9	1.06	25.8	23.6	1.09

association between socio-economic level and the status of women defined in terms of their autonomy in decision-making (see, for example, Miller 1981).

Even more interesting in Table 6.7 is the apparent role of the two processess which are traditionally believed to improve the position of women. The first and most often proposed panacea is female education. These data indicate that an educated mother certainly does experience less child loss than an uneducated one (whether one looks at boys and girls together or separately), and our results therefore belatedly confirm Caldwell's (1979) hypothesis that the education–child mortality relationship is a strong one under most circumstances. But although her capacity to increase the chances of the survival of her children seems to increase with education, the typical Uttar Pradesh woman's ability to treat her male and female offspring equally actually decreases. In other words, the advantages in preventing mortality conferred by education are being used, at least in the initial stages of the spread of education, to selectively favour boys more than girls.

But perhaps this contradiction is not so strange after all. For while the slight education, which is all that most of our literate North Indian respondents can boast of, increases their confidence and ability to improve the household physical environment and to deal with the outside world, especially the terrifying outside world of hospitals and doctors, this education hardly provides any reasons for increasing the value of girls. This is particularly the case when one considers the fact that the educated women are likely to belong to the higher socio-economic groups where the autonomy and independence of women are somewhat less than in the lower castes and classes.

And nor is this finding unique to the present study. The left half of Table 6.8 displays sex-wise rural estimates of q(5) according to maternal literacy status, derived from data from the 1981 census. The education variable we use is limited to women who are literate but have not gone up to primary schooling. This seems to be justified because (*a*) a few years of school is the most that the bulk of literate women in the country can boast, (*b*) confining the sample in this way controls to some extent for other socio-economic factors, and (*c*) even a few years of schooling has a marked impact on child mortality.

The findings from Table 6.8 are initially a little surprising.

Table 6.8. Differences in the sex ratio of childhood mortality: q(5) for males/ q(5) for females, according to maternal characteristics, rural areas

Region/state	Women's characteristics					
	Illiterate	Literate	Non-working	Working	Non-manual workers	
(1)	(2)	(3)	(4)	(5)	(6)	
All India	0.92	0.99	0.90	0.99	1.04	
North						
Haryana	0.80	0.95	0.82	0.91	1.25	
Madhya Pradesh	0.96	1.01	0.91	1.00	1.04	
Punjab	0.87	0.87	0.87	0.92	1.15	
Rajasthan	0.89	0.92	0.88	0.92	0.95	
Uttar Pradesh	0.83	0.80	0.82	0.91	0.93	
South						
Andhra Pradesh	1.05	1.14	1.07	1.04	1.15	
Karnataka	1.01	1.05	1.02	1.01	1.08	
Kerala	1.07	1.11	1.12	1.15	1.18	
Tamil Nadu	0.99	1.06	1.01	1.02	1.10	

Source: Registrar General of India (1988), *Census of India 1981: Child Mortality Estimates of India*, Government of India, New Delhi.

While there is a very distinct fall in the child mortality experience of literate mothers, there is not a consistent difference in the sex ratio of child mortality between educated and uneducated mothers for the northern region. This is also in line with the finding that juvenile sex ratios have scarcely fallen over time in this region even though female literacy rates have climbed, especially rapidly in the case of Punjab. (See also Weinberger and Heligman 1987, for a general discussion on the relationship between social and economic variables and sex differences in mortality.)

Table 6.8 also brings out the other important feature of the sex differential in child mortality in India and its potential for change. This is the regional contrast which exists in the impact of maternal education on sex differentials in child mortality and which also explains the confusion in the literature about the relationship, with some (for example, Das Gupta 1987) saying that these sex differentials are wider for educated mothers, and others (for example, Caldwell, Reddy, and Caldwell 1983) saying that they are narrower. Once the cultural context is specified (in this case the North Indian state of Punjab in the former study and the southern state of Karnataka in the latter), there is no disagreement between the two views.

All the above is certainly not to make the point that female education is an unnecessary goal. For, after all, daughter survival is higher among educated mothers, even if the increase is not as large as it is for sons. The aim here is simply to stress that the hold of culture is strong and cannot be released with simple literacy and basic education. The relevant elements of this culture are the traditional inhibitions which often make it difficult to have a girl examined, especially by a male doctor, and the conservative female life-style which limits the economic worth of women. The solution is probably to raise levels of female education significantly higher than those current in a typical poor North Indian population and to supplement the awareness and knowledge imparted by education with services, particularly in health, being made more conducive to use by women and girls, and with greater opportunities for the economic emancipation of women. Of these, the latter option seems to have strong potential as seen in the last part of Table 6.7 Maternal occupation seems to be the only variable for which both regional groups show a clear fall in the sex differential in child mortality. The mechanisms are not simple but must include the greater confidence of women with increased exposure to the outside world and the awareness that girls are also potentially economically useful individuals.

This conclusion is also supported by the macro evidence. The right half of Table 6.8 is based on rural data from the 1981 census on the sex-wise probability of death by the age of five according to whether or not the mother works. There is no ambiguity in the direction of this association. For every northern state (including the odd one out in the education case—Haryana), the sons and daughters of working mothers face more equal risks of death than the children of non-working mothers, where the relative advantage of boys is consistently greater. In some states the difference is larger than in others and we would speculate that this has something to do with the occupational mix of working women. For example, it is quite plausible that the sex ratio of childhood mortality is the most egalitarian in the case of children whose mothers work outside the home for a well-defined cash income. This is a pleasantly surprising finding because as yet we had been led to expect (from macro-level data as in Table 6.2) only that the sex differential in mortality would be smaller in areas where the potential for women's participation in the labour-force was greater (see, for example, Schultz 1982). But it now appears that even in areas with low overall female employment and probably low female employment potential as well, there is a difference in the sex ratio of child mortality between working and non-working women.

But we are now faced with another dilemma. The working mother seems to believe in equal treatment for her sons and daughters, but the overall amount and quality of this treatment is inferior to that provided by the non-working mother, so that child mortality rates are actually higher among children of employed mothers. The employment–mortality relationship has already been discussed in the previous chapter, and here we only need to add that whatever its other disadvantages, these are potentially surmountable and should be surmounted because of the one big redeeming feature of such economic independence, a significant rise in the position of women in ways which are intimately linked to their very survival, especially as daughters.

Before closing the case for the relevance of women's employment to more equal treatment of sons and daughters, one needs to consider a final confounding factor. Could it be the case that working women exhibit a more egalitarian sex ratio of child mortality not because they believe in and practise equal treatment, but because they do not have the means (in this case primarily the time and the attention) to discriminate more effectively against their daughters and in favour of their sons. This argument is analogous to the one which attributes the worse sex differential in child mortality among educated mothers to their enhanced skills in manipulating child survival. The non-working mother is, in such an analogy, comparable to the educated mother in having a greater control over her children's survival and therefore a greater ability to discriminate. For after all, overall child mortality is substantially higher among working women, as it is among the uneducated as compared to the educated. This argument can be tested by comparing the sex ratio of childhood mortality for better-off working mothers, who are able to override the negative aspects of their jobs, with that for non-working women. Column 6 of Table 6.8 does this and finds that even when mothers theoretically have the means to influence their children's survival status and when this rises markedly, the mothers who work continue to maintain a more balanced sex ratio of child mortality.

6.2. Nutritional Status

This is one area where there is almost universal lay agreement that there is active discrimination against some members of the household. However, a cold look at the evidence suggests that the case is far from clear-cut. To consider the indirect evidence first, the usual practice is to infer from the well-established sex differential in mortality, especially in childhood, that there must be and are corresponding sex differentials in feeding habits, especially in childhood. But why should we accept this inference? Malnutrition is but one of the possible precursors to death and, if recent research is to be believed, not nearly as important as originally thought. As has been pointed out in recent years (see, for example, Aaby 1988; Basu 1989), the connection is far from necessary; several other variables can explain differential mortality by sex.

Coming to the more direct evidence, Tables 6.9 and 6.10, which are based on the present study, suggest that there is little reason to believe that severe malnutrition is significantly higher in girls than in boys. Indeed it appeared in the survey that on the whole severe malnutrition was greater in the North Indian boys than in the girls, while in the Tamil Nadu case, the boys had a slight edge over girls. This result is in direct contradiction of that expected from indirect inferences in the literature. However, it should be noted that although we propose that higher levels of malnutrition do not necessarily lead to higher levels of mortality, it might still simultaneously be the case that those children who do die belong largely to the worst nourished groups. This means that the severely malnourished individuals in each age-group represent the survivors from previous age-groups and therefore, with sex or regional differentials in mortality in any age-group, the succeeding age-groups would consist of more heterogeneous populations, thereby biasing the distributional pattern of nutritional levels. This could partly explain why the proportion of severely malnourished girls in Uttar Pradesh is much smaller in all age-groups than that of males; for example, the much greater probability of dying by age 2 leaves a smaller absolute number of girls over the 0–23 months age-range as well as in the next age-group.

We attempt a (very) rough correction for such a bias below

$$\text{Uttar Pradesh girls: } q(5) = 0.259$$
$$\text{Uttar Pradesh boys: } q(5) = 0.228$$

Therefore from an initial cohort of 100 each, if girls had the same probability of dying by age five as boys, there would be $0.259 - 0.220 = 3.1$ extra girls in the 24–59 months age-group. If we make the extreme assumption that all these girls belong to the 'severe malnutrition' category, then the revised breakdown by nutritional level of the girls in the 24–59 months age-group would be as follows:

Level of malnutrition:

	Normal/mild	Moderate	Severe
Weight-for-age	41.94	47.84	10.21
Weight-for-height	61.91	32.33	5.76

Table 6.9. Nutritional classification of children by sex according to weight-for-age (%)

Region and age-group (in months)	Boys			Girls		
	Malnutrition level			Malnutrition level		
	Normal/mild	Moderate	Severe	Normal/mild	Moderate	Severe
Uttar Pradesh						
0–11	48.5	34.8	16.7	50.0	38.0	12.0
12–23	34.5	49.1	16.4	33.3	59.5	7.1
24–59	39.1	50.6	10.3	43.2	49.3	7.4
60–119	35.8	56.6	7.5	42.8	51.0	6.2
All ages	38.4	51.1	10.5	42.9	49.8	7.4
Tamil Nadu						
0–11	65.0	27.5	7.5	56.2	43.8	0.0
12–23	43.6	46.1	10.3	30.8	51.3	18.6
24–59	36.7	58.2	5.1	44.5	42.6	12.9
60–119	32.4	57.0	10.6	28.8	60.3	11.0
All ages	39.2	52.3	8.5	36.8	51.9	11.3

Sample size: Uttar Pradesh—503 boys, 434 girls; Tamil Nadu—319 boys, 318 girls.

Table 6.10. Nutritional classification of children by sex according to weight-for-height

Region and age-group (in months)	Boys			Girls		
	Malnutrition level			Malnutrition level		
	Normal/mild	Moderate	Severe	Normal/mild	Moderate	Severe
Uttar Pradesh						
0–11	76.2	12.7	11.1	60.5	27.9	11.6
12–23	49.1	43.6	7.3	51.2	41.5	7.3
24–59	57.9	36.2	5.9	63.8	33.3	2.8
60–119	49.1	46.0	4.9	53.4	42.9	3.7
All ages	55.3	38.5	6.3	57.4	38.0	4.5
Tamil Nadu						
0–11	60.0	27.5	12.3	65.5	27.6	6.9
12–23	64.9	21.6	13.5	56.8	37.8	5.4
24–59	63.4	32.3	4.3	62.9	33.0	4.1
60–119	57.7	40.0	1.5	54.3	40.6	5.1
All ages	60.7	34.0	5.3	58.5	36.5	5.0

Sample size: Uttar Pradesh—494 boys, 416 girls; Tamil Nadu—300 boys, 301 girls.

In these revised figures, the proportion of girls severely under-nourished is still lower than for boys by both the weight-for-age and weight-for-height criteria. However it must be admitted that the difference is no longer striking. But it is interesting that in spite of this correction, the girls fail to have worse nutritional levels than the boys.

We also have some (albeit approximate) data on sex differentials in actual food consumption. Since these were obtained by the method of previous day's recall by the mother, it would be unwise to set too much store by them, but the overall impression seems to be that in the Uttar Pradesh sample, girls did have a slightly better diet than boys in the case of some choice foods such as fruit and eggs (though they did somewhat worse on milk consumption), while for the Tamil sample, there was little to choose between the sexes as far as food intake was concerned. Perhaps one should add that this picture is not the result of favouritism towards girls in the northern sample but probably reflects circumstances such as a greater presence at home, which increases the access of girls to food, especially to snacks. But the researcher working with small intensive samples feels more secure if secondary data support (or at least do not contradict) the results obtained. I therefore now turn to a critical review of the existing knowledge in this area and conclude that the case in favour of the selective nutritional deprivation of girls has not been made convincingly.

To begin with the ethnographic literature, Miller (1981) did an extremely painstaking search of the literature in this context, so I think that we can assume that her evidence is the best that this literature has to offer. Her first conclusion is that the subject of sex differentials in feeding patterns has been virtually ignored by ethnographers. While this could indeed reflect a preoccupation with other topics, one wonders if the scant attention is at least partly because field researchers have found so little to report: one hopes that the anthropologist who sees consistent underfeeding of girls *vis-à-vis* boys in a society would find this sufficiently interesting to explore. The argument here is similar to Miller's argument that since the anthropological literature on North India is replete with descriptions about the joy experienced at the birth of a son while that on South India is not, this means that such excessive joy is less present in the South.

The result is that although Miller (1981) devotes much more

space to feeding differentials by sex than to differentials in health care, she is on much weaker ground in the former case. For example, the evidence on breast-feeding is at best inconclusive, especially since differentials in the duration of breast-feeding can affect both nutrition and mortality in either direction, depending on the circumstances. For instance, the (slightly) younger age at which girls have the *annaprasan* ceremony (which marks the introduction of solid foods) in some parts of India could mean that there is a greater hurry to get them off the breast though it must also be mentioned that all that this ceremony heralds is the cessation of total breast-feeding; partial breast-feeding continues), but its practical result may well be that girls now get a more balanced diet than boys. For example, in the Morinda study, Levinson (1972) found that in upper-caste households, fully weaned girls and semi-weaned boys showed little difference in total nutrient intake.

The possibility of so many interpretations means that the mother suspected of discriminating against her daughters in food often faces a no-win situation (for example, see Pettigrew 1986); if the daughter is breast-fed longer than the son, it is because the mother (or parents, or grandmother) does not want to spend money on other food; if she is breast-fed for a shorter while, it is because breastmilk is considered more important for boys.

The other major kind of evidence, used by Miller and others to support the hypothesis of better feeding of boys than of girls in northern India in particular and South Asia in general, relies on statements about choice foods (the most common one being *ghee* or clarified butter) being preferentially given to sons. Some researchers (for example, Khan *et al.* 1988; Gupta 1985; Das Gupta 1987) also report some direct evidence on this score. In our own study, in 13 per cent of the Uttar Pradesh homes, the boys ate meat and eggs while the girls did not (the male–female difference was even greater for adults); in the Tamil sample there was no such household. But while this discrimination would be likely to lead to greater (and surely unhealthy) obesity in boys if carried on to a sufficient extreme, this does not really warrant the conclusion that girls are worse fed in the net result, especially since choice foods form such a small part of the total diet of the typical South Asian household. Moreover, it should be noted that parents who say that they reserve the special food for boys are also likely to say that they do not discriminate in the allocation of more ordinary food (for example, Chen, Huq, and D'Souza, 1981; Khan *et al.* 1988). However, it must be admitted that such statements about and actual reservation of choice foods does say something about household attitudes towards boys and girls and towards their separate needs. Finally, the anthropological studies from South India which describe the fine food given to girls at menarche should really be treated more as the observation of a ritual than overall preferential feeding of girls over boys.

There are other pitfalls in giving too much weight to such descriptive or anecdotal evidence, the main one being the problem of biased samples. This is well illustrated in Pettigrew (1986), where the author talks of the positive discrimination towards a son and the negative discrimination against the youngest daughter in a family with one son and four daughters. But this is surely an atypical case and in the kind of poor household she is describing, one suspects that the youngest would suffer even if he were male, in a family with four sons and one daughter. That is, there is a birth-order effect and a sex-composition effect firmly entangled in the sex-preference effect we are concerned with.

Coming to more quantitative findings, the evidence is once more not as unequivocal as it appears at first glance or as it would appear if one went by a WHO review of the area (World Health Organization 1986). Footnote 1 on p. 2 of this review gives away the biased stand from which it proceeds: 'studies cited in this review are thus by definition limited mainly to those that have found evidence of discrimination; studies that have found no such differences are therefore not mentioned here.' Apparently, this has been done to 'convey a sense of urgency of the problem'. The logic of this attitude is puzzling; you can hardly point to the gravity of, say, a water shortage in a region by singling out the six homes with no water and ignoring the dozens that have more than they know what to do with.

To take the quantitative evidence on breast-feeding first, most studies report no significant sex differentials in duration (for example, Wyon and Gordon 1971; Huffman *et al.* 1980). Jain and Bongaarts (1981), in an analysis of World Fertility Survey data from eight countries (including Bangladesh, where sex differentials in mortality are high), found no evidence of longer duration of breast-feeding for boys than for girls. This is in spite of the fact that there is some suggestion in the literature that birth intervals are shorter after a girl than after a boy; in fact, this finding is used to infer (wrongly, as it appears from more direct data) shorter breast-feeding for girls. In any case, it must be stated that even if sex differentials in breast-feeding did exist, it would be difficult to know how to interpret their connection with final nutritional levels.

The mean lengths of breast-feeding in our field study are displayed in Table 6.11. I present durations separately for all live births in the last ten years, and current survivors of all live births in the last ten years. Children under the age of one are not included in the calculations of mean breast-feeding duration because so many of them fall in the category of 'still breast-feeding', as seen in the last two columns of the table. It is interesting to note that, contrary to expectations, it is among the Tamils that sex differences in breast-feeding are more heavily weighted against girls.

Next, there are field surveys which take anthropometric measurements and classify them with reference to a standard such as the Harvard. There is a potential problem here. Might it be more realistic to use different cut-off points for girls and boys

Table 6.11. Mean length of breast-feeding
by region and sex of child

Region and months since birth	All live births		Only living children			
					% Still Continuing	
	Boys	Girls	Boys	Girls	Boys	Girls
Uttar Pradesh						
0–11					99.2	98.0
12–59	17.8	18.8	19.9	19.5	40.0	36.3
60–119	21.8	21.5	25.1	24.4		
Tamil Nadu						
0–11					97.8	81.8
12–59	13.8	15.0	15.3	16.0	59.9	81.8
60–119	20.0	16.7	21.9	18.7		

Note. Cases still breast-feeding were excluded when calculating the means in cols. 2–5.

Sample size. Uttar Pradesh—all live births, 554 boys, 402 girls; living children, 542 boys, 452 girls; Tamil Nadu—all live births, 364 boys, 360 girls; living children, 351 boys, 344 girls.

while determining nutritional levels? In the South Asian context, this could well be appropriate, given the greater seclusion of girls and their lesser involvement in activities which consume energy, especially in the pre-adolescent stages. Another problem with the interpretation of findings from field studies based on anthropometric measurements is that malnutrition levels reported for the two sexes in several such surveys may be biased by the choice of reference standard. Fore example, although Sen and Sengupta (1983) and Kielmann and associates (1983) report a higher incidence of severe malnutrition in girls than in boys, they seem not to have used sex-specific reference tables for classifying their observations. And the fact is that even the Harvard and National Centre for Health Statistics standards commonly employed have girls displaying lower median heights and weights than boys of the same age, and I do not think anyone would argue that there is food discrimination against girls in the populations from which these standards are derived.

I illustrate the relevance of a sex-specific standard by reclassifying the data on which Tables 6.9 and 6.10 are based, now using the sex-independent growth chart developed at the Institute of Health and Nutrition, Delhi, which is based on the Harvard standards and now recommended for use in the field by health-workers in India. The results are set out in Table 6.12. The changed picture (as compared with Tables 6.9 and 6.10) is striking. No longer can we confidently assert that girls from Uttar Pradesh exhibit better nutritional status than boys. In fact, for most of the age-groups and for both measures (weight-for-age as well as weight-for-height), it is now the girls that seem more severely deprived. And in the Tamil sample, the earlier relatively small disadvantage to girls is much sharper now.

On the other hand, it is true that the choice of reference standard can affect the bias in the opposite direction as well. For example, using an Indian sex-specific standard derived from children from well-to-do homes in Hyderabad, the Indian National Institute of Nutrition (1984) found that in six of the seven states for which it had anthropometric data for children, boys were decidedly worse off than girls. However, as Gopalan (1987) has pointed out, the Hyderabad standard itself is biased, setting much lower standards than do the National Centre for Health Statistics and Harvard standards (this may be more realistic in the Indian

Table 6.12. Nutritional classification of children using a sex-independent weight-for-age standard

Region and age-group (in months)	Boys			Girls		
	Malnutrition level			Malnutrition level		
	Normal/mild	Moderate	Severe	Normal/mild	Moderate	Severe
Uttar Pradesh						
0–11	53.1	31.3	15.6	40.0	38.0	22.0
12–23	33.9	44.6	21.4	25.0	50.0	25.0
24–59	33.3	53.2	13.5	27.9	59.9	12.2
All ages	30.0	46.4	15.6	30.0	53.6	46.4
Tamil Nadu						
0–11	65.0	27.5	7.5	50.1	29.0	12.9
12–23	30.0	53.6	15.4	17.5	55.0	27.5
24–59	33.7	60.0	6.3	37.3	40.0	14.7
All ages	40.2	51.2	8.6	36.4	46.3	17.4

Sample: As in Table 6.9.

context), and also displaying much larger sex differentials in the mean weight-for-age and height-for-age values than these conventional standards. Reclassifying the same data using the NCHS standard, Gopalan found that the observed bias against boys disappeared. But, for our present purposes, what is more instructive is that a clear nutritional disadvantage to girls did not appear. What the data from these states in India instead show is that there is no significant evidence of a greater nutritional disadvantage in either sex. This absence of clear gender differentials in childhood nutritional levels has also come out in several other studies (see, for example, Chaudhury 1984; Chaudhury 1987; Nutrition Foundation of India 1988; Visaria 1988) and once it becomes less awkward to take this neutral stand, perhaps more such studies will gain publicity.

But there is at least one study which used sex-specific standards to classify its anthropometric measurements and still found greater malnutrition in girls than in boys in Matlab *thana* (an administrative area of about 200 000 persons) in Bangladesh (see Chen 1982). Moreover, an equally careful study in one sub-sample of this project even found that females received less food than males (Chen, Huq, and D'Souza 1981). While it may be difficult to fault these findings on methodological grounds, one should consider the author's cautionary note (Chen 1982) that the findings might not be generalizable to other parts of South Asia.

In fact, it is worth noting that once the above food-intake study had been corrected for sex differences in dietary requirements based on body mass, physical activity, and the special needs of the female reproductive cycle, it was only for the 0–4 years age-group that it could be said with any definiteness that the shortfall in food intake was greater for girls than for boys (which probably means only the 1–4 years group in reality, since breast-feeding is near universal and total in the first year of life in these parts). Unfortunately this part of their finding has received considerably less attention than their demonstration of greater discrimination against girls in early childhood.

The little other evidence we have on sex differences in the intra-household distribution of food is again mixed (for summaries of this evidence, see Harris 1990 and Lipton 1983). Two important points emerge repeatedly. The first is that the more relevant distinction is probably that between children and adults (although even the interpretation of the fact of greater malnourishment among children has problems given the over-representation of children among the poor, that is, among the malnourished; see Lipton 1983), rather than boys *vis-à-vis* girls. However, in our study, we found that only in a small percentage of cases were children not likely to be among the first family members to be fed (see Table 5.9 in the previous chapter). But there was also a regional differential in this and in households from the southern state of Tamil Nadu, children were given first preference in virtually all cases.

Secondly, it appears that where actual discrimination against girls does exist, it is more likely to begin in late childhood or early adolescence as the girl is socialized for the role of ideal wife and mother (for Bangladesh, see Rizvi 1983). In India too, Appadurai (1981) records that any sex discrimination in the gastro-political roles prescribed for boys and girls tends to start at about age 5. But even at these older ages, anthropometric data are increasingly beginning to suggest that we may be making an unduly strong case in favour of a female disadvantage; the actual evidence (see, for example, Nutrition Foundation of India 1988; Gopalan 1987; Chaudhury 1987) strongly suggests that food imbalances are not a major part of the gender inequalities in South Asia.

6.3. Health Status

This area of physical welfare is obviously related to the findings in earlier sections on intra-household differences in mortality and nutritional level. But, for one thing, intra-household mortality and nutritional differentials are not necessarily in the same direction. More importantly, one's state of health is also independently determined by a series of variables not directly related to mortality rates or nutritional status. For example, we have the recent conclusion from the Centre for Development Studies, Trivandrum, that in spite of very favourable mortality conditions in Kerala, morbidity or sickness levels may be much higher in this state than in other parts of the country (Pannikar and Soman 1984).

From the perspective of intra-family differences in health, one can look at differences in two categories of influences: those which influence exposure to an illness and those which influence the outcome of an illness. In the former category I look at gender differences in life-styles as they affect health and in preventive medical care, that is, immunization. In the latter category I consider differences in health-care-seeking behaviour once an illness has occurred. Differences in health care use can lead to differences in mortality at one extreme, of course; in addition, they can be responsible for differences in overall health status by directly affecting the severity and duration of an illness.

Life-styles

In both childhood and adulthood, one can easily see that certain kinds of life-styles increase the risk of exposure to disease more than others. For example, there is the health impact of smoking, which is believed to be a major culprit in the narrowing sex differential in adult mortality in the Western world; with more and more women taking to cigarettes, they are losing the advantage in life expectancy that they have traditionally had over men.

More relevantly to the Indian context, in childhood, differentials in school attendance or in income-earning activities can conceivably add new risk factors to the lives of some members of the family. However, such differences in activity are rare in the very young, that is, among the under-5s, and even in older children they tend to be in favour of girls. For example, in the present study, the girls from Uttar Pradesh were less likely to go to school than the boys and, given the overcrowding and unhygienic conditions in the local schools, this means that the boys faced a greater risk of infection. This may account for the slightly higher incidence of illness in boys in the study (although one can never completely rule out the role of differential reporting of illness; sickness in boys has a tendency to cause a faster reaction in terms of recognition and action than in the case of girls).

But more invidious in its impact on health than the incidence of an illness is the severity of the illness episode. And here, recent evidence from Senegal and Bangladesh (see Aaby 1988) suggests that differences in life-styles are more disadvantageous to girls. For example, it appears to be quite well confirmed in the above research that the severity of an infectious illness is affected by the intensity of exposure, which in the traditional South Asian context is likely to be greater for girls. This is because girls are more likely to stay at home and therefore more likely to become what are known as secondary cases, that is, cases that have become infected from another household member as opposed to index or primary cases which have been exposed to infection from a relative outsider such as a school companion. Since one spends more time with other household members (just consider the hours of sleep every night) than with outsiders, it is postulated that secondary cases face a greater intensity of exposure and thus severity of infection. This kind of reasoning partly explains why infections tend to be more fatal in the very young (who are almost always secondary cases), the very old, and, in our kind of set-up, girls, because the fewer restrictions on the movement of boys increase their chances of contracting an illness outside the home.

Gender differences in life-style are also responsible for the rapidly increasing risk of ill-health in young males from accidents and injuries, and most studies all over the world on violence as a source of ill-health and death confirm the higher vulnerability of this age- and sex-group. Of course, I am excluding the balancing effect in some parts of India of deaths or trauma by violence in the case of young married persons accused of not satisfying material demands; for these the order of vulnerability according to sex is completely reversed. I am also excluding the great sex imbalance in aborted foetuses when the abortions follow the increasingly popular amniocentesis procedure for determination of the sex of the foetus.

Finally, one should mention the selective adverse impact on women's health of childbearing, which it is true cannot be passed on to men, but which can nevertheless be considerably reduced by lowered fertility and better health care, and secondly by their disproportionate responsibility for household contraceptive practice (for a detailed discussion of this issue, see Basu 1985).

Preventive Health Care

On the whole, it appears that there are no important gender differences in prophylactic health care or immunization acceptance. For example, in our sample, there were very small sex differences in the percentage of living children who had received some immunization (although there were interesting regional differences as was discussed in the last chapter). This absence of a marked sex differential in immunization has been confirmed by the all-India survey of infant and child mortality conducted by the Registrar General of India (1981*a*). However, it should be noted that the immunization status of living children may present a distorted picture. This may be why we found that when all live births were considered, girls fared markedly worse, especially for Uttar Pradesh. On the other hand this latter finding could also mean that the girls had died before they could be immunized, so the direction of causality is not at all clear. But on the whole it does appear that preventive measures are not sex selective (witness also, for example, the lack of a sex differential in the incidence of even those diseases preventable by immunization; see Chen 1982), and this is not surprising because immunization is generally a one-shot procedure and one where girls can be easily taken along with boys, unlike in the case of illness where each bout represents a separate event which cannot be handled in combination with other events.

Curative Health Care

We come finally to the possibility of gender differences in the treatment of illness. How strong is this possibility? To begin with, Singh, Gordon, and Wyon (1962) found that children under 3 years, females, and low-caste groups had less and lower quality medical care than the remainder in the Khanna Study in Punjab. These were also the groups with the highest death-rates. The female disadvantage in survival was especially sharp in children less than 2 years old; girls died from the same causes as boys, their mothers started them on solid food at the same age as boys, but the parents gave boys higher-quality medical care. Similarly, in the Matlab area in Bangladesh, where free treatment of diarrhoeal diseases was offered to the entire study population, it was found that in spite of nearly comparable incidence levels of .diarrhoeas between boys and girls, male children were far more likely than females to be brought to the treatment facility by their guardians (Chen, Huq, and D'Souza, 1981); visits for male children aged 0–4 years were 66 per cent higher than for female children, and male children were also about twice as likely to be hospitalized for treatment as female children. Aziz's (1977) study of medical care prior to fatal illness in Bangladesh confirmed that girls were less likely to have received medical care and less likely to have received competent medical care than boys.

Table 6.13 reports the findings of our survey on sex differentials in the handling of morbid episodes based on the illnesses reported in the six-month longitudinal study. As in Chapter 5, we concentrate on four of the most commonly occurring groups of illnesses: fevers, respiratory ailments, gastro-intestinal ailments, and skin disorders. The first noticeable feature of Table 6.13 is the sex bias in the proportions of children receiving no treatment; girls are much more likely to fall into this category than boys. However, there are clear regional differentials in the nature of this sex bias. The most striking is the fact that although the sex differential is the greatest in the treatment of fever, in the two regional groups the direction of this bias is diametrically opposite. The role of fever as a particularly incapacitating and worrying ailment has been discussed in the previous chapter. What is unusual is the finding that while fever is the illness most likely to be treated by the Uttar Pradesh households, it is also the illness where the disadvantage of girls *vis-à-vis* boys is the greatest. On the other hand, for the South Indian sample, there seems to be a much greater urgency to do something about a fever if the sufferer happens to be a girl. However, the possibility must be admitted that this is less because of an emotional bias towards daughters than because of the greater opportunity costs of an inactivating illness such as fever in girls, since the girls from Tamil Nadu were much more involved both in housework (especially if their mothers worked) as well as in income-earning activities outside the home (even in the 5–9 years age-group).

But to analyse further the regional influences on sex differentials in treatment one needs to go beyond a simple treatment/no treatment dichotomous variable. The kind of treatment is as important a determinant as the fact of treatment; indeed it is often more important because some kinds of treatment are no better than or sometimes even worse than no treatment at all. In the present survey, the last category of 'other methods' of treatment represents one such group, which is important not only because it is often virtually ineffective but also because resort to this group (which is essentially made up of mainly traditional and some

Table 6.13. The handling of children's illness episodes according to region of origin, type of illness, age, and sex

Region and nature of illness	Age-group (in years)	% Receiving the following treatment									
		None		Government doctor		Private doctor		Modern home remedy		Others	
		Boys	Girls	Boys	Girls	Boys	Girls	Boys	Girls	Boys	Girls
Uttar Pradesh											
Fever	< 5	3.9	8.9	23.9	21.4	80.8	75.0	2.3	4.5	0.0	0.0
	5–9	6.6	12.3	14.5	28.1	84.2	68.4	2.6	1.8	0.0	3.5
Respiratory illness	< 5	18.2	19.3	12.2	15.9	69.1	55.2	3.3	7.6	4.4	3.4
	5–9	16.8	15.0	12.2	18.3	66.4	63.3	8.4	8.3	1.9	5.0
Gastro-intestinal illness	< 5	14.4	14.1	19.5	14.9	73.9	73.6	1.0	3.3	2.6	5.0
	5–9	20.9	9.7	18.6	16.1	69.8	64.5	0.0	3.2	4.7	12.9
Skin disease	< 5	20.4	18.2	17.5	19.7	51.5	59.1	5.8	9.1	1.9	6.1
	5–9	18.9	8.9	23.0	31.1	54.1	68.9	8.1	2.2	8.2	2.2
Tamil Nadu											
Fever	< 5	18.9	11.1	16.2	11.1	64.9	75.0	5.4	5.6	0.0	2.8
	5–9	18.2	10.7	9.1	21.4	57.6	57.1	18.2	10.7	0.0	0.0
Respiratory illness	< 5	11.1	21.1	10.0	8.9	78.9	66.7	3.3	4.4	1.1	1.1
	5–9	25.0	27.1	15.6	6.4	40.6	52.1	21.9	14.6	0.0	0.0
Gastro-intestinal illness	< 5	7.5	22.8	25.0	15.8	72.5	64.9	0.0	1.8	5.0	0.0
	5–9	20.0	0.0	20.0	0.0	40.0	100.0	20.0	0.0	0.0	0.0
Skin disease	< 5	16.7	10.7	12.5	14.3	62.5	71.4	8.3	3.6	0.0	3.6
	5–9	18.2	9.1	0.0	0.0	54.6	72.7	9.1	13.6	18.2	4.6

Notes:
Total number of illnesses = Uttar Pradesh: 1546; Tamil Nadu: 583.
The percentages add up to more than 100 because some illnesses received more than one kind of treatment.

modern home remedies) constitutes the line of least effort and cost and therefore is a reflection of the importance given to an illness. And once more, consistently with our other data, it is the boys from Uttar Pradesh who are considered least likely to benefit from such self-medication. The first part of Table 6.14 presents sex differentials in the proportion of illnesses receiving non-professional treatment (that is, the sum of cases getting no treatment, home remedies, and 'other' treatments). The regional contrast is now sharper. Except for skin diseases in the 5–9 years age-group, in every single case the North Indian girls are thought much less deserving of treatment or at best deserving of non-professional treatment than the boys. For the Tamil sample, however, there is no clear picture; if anything, the boys do worse than the girls more often than vice-versa.

This brings us to the use of western or modern curative medicine. Since girls did better than boys in the combined category of 'no treatment' and 'other treatment', it follows that they show lower rates for the use of modern clinical medicine. And whatever its other faults, the ability of such treatment to ward off death in the short run is well known. But even more interesting is the kind of medical practitioner that is favoured. As discussed in the previous chapters, our data indicate a uniform tendency to consider the private practitioner to be superior to the government one, even though the services of the latter are free. And given the trend of our findings from Tables 6.13 and 6.14 so far, it is therefore not surprising that the boys from Uttar Pradesh are more likely to visit a private clinic than the girls (see the last column in Table 6.14), while in the Tamil Nadu case, once more the results are mixed. There are two more implications of this pattern of health care use: the treatment of illness in girls is more likely to be delayed to avoid the long wait at the government clinic and, secondly, the greater willingness to spend money on the treatment of sons again reflects the relatively greater importance given to an illness episode in a son.

I would suggest that besides affecting the general state of health, this difference in the amount and kind of medical care provided during illness is an important determinant of the sex differences in child mortality observed in our North Indian sample and, indeed, in several contemporary populations in which girls face a disadvantage in survival.

Table 6.14. Distribution of children's illness episodes receiving professional modern medical treatment by region of origin, type of illness, age and sex

Region and nature of illness	Age-group (in years)	% of cases getting non-professional or no treatment		% of cases getting modern professional treatment		% of professionally seen cases attended by a private doctor	
		Boys	Girls	Boys	Girls	Boys	Girls
Uttar Pradesh							
Fever	< 5	6.2	13.4	104.7	96.4	77.2	77.8
	5–9	9.2	17.6	98.7	96.5	85.3	70.9
Respiratory illness	< 5	25.9	30.3	81.3	71.1	85.0	77.6
	5–9	27.1	28.3	78.6	81.6	84.5	77.6
Gastro-intestinal illness	< 5	18.0	22.4	93.4	88.5	79.1	83.2
	5–9	25.6	25.8	88.4	88.6	79.0	80.0
Skin disease	< 5	28.1	33.4	69.0	78.8	74.6	75.0
	5–9	35.2	13.3	77.1	100.0	70.2	68.9
Tamil Nadu							
Fever	< 5	24.3	19.5	81.1	86.1	80.0	87.1
	5–9	36.4	21.4	66.7	78.5	86.4	72.1
Respiratory illness	< 5	15.5	26.6	88.9	75.6	88.8	88.2
	5–9	46.9	41.7	56.2	58.4	72.2	89.2
Gastro-intestinal illness	< 5	12.5	24.6	97.5	80.7	74.4	80.4
	5–9	40.0	0.0	60.8	100.0	66.7	100.0
Skin disease	< 5	25.0	17.9	75.0	85.7	83.3	83.3
	5–9	45.5	27.3	54.6	72.7	100.0	100.0

Note: Total number of illnesses = Uttar Pradesh: 1546; Tamil Nadu: 583.

6.4. Discussion

If the last several pages have a message, it is that the picture has too many shades of grey, especially now, with trends in intra-household differences in physical welfare moving in directions which are not always consistent. For example, while the sex ratio of infant mortality in India seems to be nearing unity, it seems to be increasing in a direction against males for mortality in young adults. Similarly, while health-care use tends to favour boys and men, nutritional levels may be better in girls and women. It is important to note these distinctions because, by painting the picture an unrelieved black, one only ends up diverting attention away from those issues on which sex differences are relevant and more urgently in need of attention.

How does the position of women fit into these descriptions of sex differences in physical well-being? In several ways, both direct and indirect. The first revealing finding of course is that there are clear North–South differences in gender inequalities especially in survival, even when we try to keep socio-economic circumstances constant, just as there are clear North–South differences in the position of women even when socio-economic conditions are similar. But why should there be a connection between these two findings? One can group the hypothesized intermediate variables responsible for such a connection into two broad categories of behaviour:

(*a*) custom or unconscious behaviour which is unrelated to a deliberate discrimination against one sex; and

(*b*) behaviour based on a conscious valuation of one sex over the other.

The two need to be distinguished because the intervention points to affect them can also be different.

To recall Chapter 3, the discussion on marriage systems and women's employment opportunities stressed the great regional difference that exists in the seclusion norms for women and in their economic dependence on men. Both these features lead to a devaluation of women at least in the economic sense and perhaps in other areas of life as well. Or, if one were to sound less harsh and still convey the same meaning, they lead to a much higher value being attached to the male. In a situation of limited resources, this often translates into a gender differential in

resource allocation. The rationales for such an unbalanced allocation of resources can be viewed in two complementary ways. The
first is a smaller investment in girls than in boys in North India
because girls are seen as potentially less crucial for family welfare;
in extreme cases they may even by viewed as positively detrimental to family welfare. Or alternatively, to continue the more
charitable style of interpretation, it is vital for the lives and
well-being of boys to be protected if the household is to survive
and prosper. Such investment-based interpretations have been
applied in several attempts to understand the warped sex ratio of
child mortality in the South Asian region (see, in particular,
Schultz 1982, and the section on 'Son Preference' in Chapter 4
above).

Somewhat different in their emphasis are writers such as Sen
(1987) who have argued that gender inequalities within a household are a special case of the situation of 'co-operative conflict' that
characterizes most relationships. This is the coexistence of conflict
and common interests in most forms of human interaction. The
outcomes of such situations of co-operative conflict will depend
on several factors, one important one being differences between
the parties involved in the cost of a 'breakdown' in co-operation.
The more vulnerable an agent in the event of a breakdown, the
more he or she has a vested interest in accepting a less than
satisfactory situation.

Several social, economic and cultural factors can affect the
vulnerability of women in such 'bargaining contracts' between the
sexes. One such factor which seems to stand out in our data, and
in secondary data from regions well beyond South Asia reviewed
in Drèze and Sen (1990) is the gainful employment of women. It
seems to consistently be the case that, at the macro-level, sex
differences in mortality, for example, are less marked in areas
where female labour-force participation rates are high (Bardhan,
1974). At the micro-level too, the sex ratio of child mortality is
closest to unity for women who are employed; even maternal
education does not seem to have such a distinct relationship.

It is not clear from these results whether it is the investment
mechanism or the bargaining mechanism that is at work. Some
support for the former is gained from the fact that we find sex
differentials in child mortality; presumably children are not
themselves in a position to co-operate or refuse to play the game.

Our data do not really look at sex differentials in welfare at the older ages, when co-operative conflicts are more likely to become apparent. Active discrimination against the female sex is probably derived from a combination of both kinds of motivation.

In the context of sex differentials in child mortality, the practical manifestation of both kinds of motivation is that when son preference is high and resources are fixed and low, panicky investment in the well-being of boys often means a withdrawal of much needed resources from girls. Such relative under-investment in girls is less common in a culture where women are economically active: first, because women do not need sons to improve their position in the bargaining contract when they have their own incomes to fall back on; and secondly, because women and men need to distinguish less between sons and daughters as potential sources of economic support when both sexes have access to employment.

The other important finding is the role of women's activities that are 'perceived' to be economically valuable. It is not enough to demonstrate objectively that women in any culture do not enjoy leisure but perform a range of often backbreaking tasks in addition to their domestic maintenance activities. The crucial factor seems to be whether there are recognizable material returns from this work.

The third interesting finding in this relationship between women's employment and sex differentials in welfare is that the potential for women's employment is almost as important as the fact of employment itself. This is reflected, for example, in the result that in areas of high labour-force participation rates by women, even in homes where women do not work boys and girls have relatively equal life-chances. Indeed, given the higher child mortality experience of poor working women documented in an earlier chapter, probably the best-placed mother is one who does not work herself but knows that there are no restrictions on her finding or accepting work should the need arise.

If women's employment is an important determinant of sex differentials in physical welfare, culture is influential via the norms about female employment. Employment opportunities themselves can only gradually erode such norms, as is seen in the vast regional differential in female employment in the present study, even though both groups face the same employment choices in principle.

To return to the intermediate variables in the relationship between women's status and sex differentials in well-being, we have so far been talking of direct or intentional effects, however subconscious or institutionalized the intent. But there is also an important indirect route that links these two variables of interest. This is the influence of women's status on behaviours detrimental to the well-being of the female sex even where there exists no desire to discriminate. For instance, Khan *et al.* (1988) have recorded that in their village study in Uttar Pradesh, if women did agree to go to a male doctor, they preferred to go to one in the city who did not know them rather than to one in the village who might recognize them. Given the inconveniences involved in such behaviour, the doctor is thus more likely to be the last resort for ill women than he is for ill men. Similarly, Section 6.3 above demonstrated that there were clear North–South differences in the use of modern health-care services by boys and girls, with girls from the North Indian sample having to be content more often than boys with no treatment or with non-professional treatment for a variety of ailments. At least a part of this apparent discrimination is attributable to traditional inhibitions rather than an active desire to discriminate.

Restrictions on the movements of girls and women also reinforce sex differences in health and mortality because females, who are more likely to remain at home, are also more likely as a consequence of such seclusion to become what Aaby (1988) has called secondary cases of infection than are their brothers or husbands. This means that they are more likely to become infected from another household member than from a relative outsider. This also means that their infections are likely to be more severe because of the greater dose (in terms of time) of infection that they are exposed to.

As the last chapter discusses, such indirect mechanisms are not to be taken lightly, if only because they offer hope that there are some immediate successes that practical policy methods can achieve. The interventions required to overcome these indirect effects of female status on sex differences in care can (without the heroic efforts needed to change the direct all-consuming preference for and dependence on sons) be mitigated by services that are able to bypass traditional inhibitions. One can think of more sex-segregated educational and sanitary facilities and more health centres with female staff as a very useful first step in this direction.

Our model of the relationship between the status of women and the sex differential in child mortality (as a proxy for sex differentials in physical well-being in general) would therefore be as illustrated in Fig. 6.1.

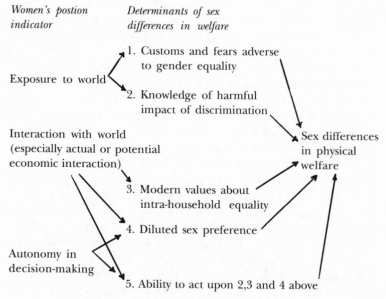

*Women's postion
indicator*

*Determinants of sex
differences in welfare*

Exposure to world

1. Customs and fears adverse to gender equality
2. Knowledge of harmful impact of discrimination

Interaction with world (especially actual or potential economic interaction)

Sex differences in physical welfare

3. Modern values about intra-household equality

4. Diluted sex preference

Autonomy in decision-making

5. Ability to act upon 2,3 and 4 above

F IG. 6.1. A model of the status of women and regional sex differences in physical welfare

Once again, as in the child mortality and fertility case, one can see that each of the women's status factors also has strong indirect effects through its influence on the other women's status variables. The largest number of arrows radiate from the variable of women's interaction (which really refers here primarily to economic interaction), especially if one includes the effect in turn of such interaction on both exposure and autonomy. The reader is referred to Chapter 7 for one final word in favour of women's increased economic relationship with the outside world.

7

Conclusions

In recent times, there has been an increasing interest in two important possible determinants of demographic behaviour: cultural background and the 'status' of women. Concern with the former variable has led to the development of what is called 'regional demography'. This is seen, for example, in the elaboration of North–South differentials in demographic indices in India, in the various analyses of fertility and mortality differences by factors such as religion and language, and in historical studies of population change that have been struck by the role of geographic factors in explaining the demographic transition. Concern with the second variable, that is, the status of women, is reflected in the scores of studies linking status-of-women indicators such as education and employment to indicators of demographic behaviour.

This book has tried to combine these two strands of research interest to conclude that cultural background in fact influences demographic behaviour in large measure through its intermediate influence on the position of women. 'Culture' was defined in terms of region of origin and cultural norms were defined as attitudes and practices common to well-defined regional groups in spite of socio-economic differences within such groups. Alternatively, such norms can be studied (as was done here) by looking at differences in attitudes and practices that exist between well-defined regional groups even when their socio-economic circumstances are held constant. The 'status of women' was defined at three levels: the extent of women's exposure to the outside world; the extent of their active (especially economic) interaction with this extra-domestic world; and their level of autonomy in decision-making. Demographic behaviour was defined to include fertility, child mortality, and sex differentials in physical well-being.

Using such definitions and a North India–South India comparison with field data as well as secondary data, I have tried to demonstrate two propositions:

(*a*) that cultural context is an important determinant of demographic behaviour; and

(*b*) the position of women is an important component of cultural background responsible for this effect.

In addition an attempt was made to identify the intermediate behavioural variables connecting women's status to demographic behaviour.

7.1. Overview of Findings

An empirical demonstration of the above propositions was attempted by a field study of two culturally distinct groups, one North Indian and the other South Indian, both living in the same locality, so that the external environment, both physical as well as in terms of access to facilities, was controlled. In addition, all the sample households belonged to the lowest socio-economic groups so that we were also able to exclude the unwanted influence of class and social status.

The focus was on three demographic variables: fertility, child mortality, and sex differences in child health and mortality. Data collection involved detailed interviews with heads of households, and with all the ever-married women in these households. In addition, during the six-month longitudinal study which followed the retrospective data collection, households with at least two living children below the age of 12 were visited once a fortnight to gather information on these children's activities, consumption patterns, illnesses, and treatment during the last two weeks.

The analysis of the data so obtained revealed the same kind of regional differences in demographic behaviour as are seen in secondary sources of information from the two states, Uttar Pradesh and Tamil Nadu, from which our two groups of respondents hailed. The Tamil women had distinctly lower levels of fertility and child mortality and a much smaller sex differential in childhood mortality than the women from Uttar Pradesh. The regional difference in this last variable was particularly striking; not only did the Tamil households not display the typical South Asian pattern of a greater female disadvantage in survival, girls actually often fared better than boys in this group. On the other hand, in the North Indian sample, at least 115 girls (even this figure is likely to be an underestimate) had died for every 100 boys that had died. The other interesting and somewhat surprising result was that this sex differential was wider for households of higher socio-economic status defined by indicators such as caste and income and even by the supposedly beneficial indicator of maternal education. This widening of the sex differential with an increase in household and (especially) maternal resources means that the advantages in preventing mortality conferred by these resources are being used, at least in the initial stages of a rise in socio-economic status, to selectively favour boys over girls. In fact, the only variable for which both regional groups showed a clear fall in the sex ratio of child mortality was the variable of maternal occupation. The reasons for this relationship are not simple, but must include the greater confidence and independence of women with increased exposure to the outside world and the awareness that girls are also potentially economically useful individuals.

As for the proximate determinants through which these sex differences in childhood mortality operate, our study concluded that the main determinant is a sex differential in the handling of illness episodes: North Indian boys are much more likely to receive modern, professional, privately obtained (that is, paid for) medical care than their sisters, and are also more likely to receive more than one bout of treatment for the same illness. Nowhere was this brought home more clearly than in the sex ratio of child deaths during the six-month longitudinal study: the Uttar Pradesh sample showed a tragically high ratio (females/males) of 8.2 for child death rates while for Tamil Nadu this index reached unity.

Then there was the clear regional difference in fertility. Chapter 4 concluded that both cumulative and current fertility were lower in the Tamil households than in those from Uttar Pradesh. Moreover, these fertility differentials were caused by an earlier halt to childbearing by the Tamil women (primarily by sterilization but also by the greater use of effective non-terminal contraception) rather than by regional differences in inter-birth intervals. Longer breast-feeding in the Uttar Pradesh households tended to be balanced by greater contraceptive use in those from Tamil Nadu. The only birth interval which varied strongly between the two groups was the first one, that is, the gap between effective marriage and the first live birth. An attempt was made to link this regional difference in the first birth interval to regional differences in marriage practices, in particular to the rules governing village exogamy. It appeared that these practices had the (possibly unintentional) side-effect of reducing exposure to the risk of pregnancy during the first few years of marriage among the northern Indians. But the shorter first birth interval for the South Indian women was balanced by the earlier age at effective marriage for the North Indian women, so that both groups eventually had very similar ages at first live birth. Moreover, socio-economic differentials in fertility were smaller for the Tamil group and regional differences in fertility were maintained within each socio-economic category.

Finally, on the issue of overall child mortality, the homes from Tamil Nadu scored better than those from Uttar Pradesh, with 111 children from the latter having died for every 100 children from the southern sample that had died. The pattern of socio-economic differentials in childhood mortality also varied greatly in the two groups: in general socio-economic differentials in child death rates were much lower for the Tamil women and also, within each socio-economic category the Tamil Nadu child death rate was consistently lower than the Uttar Pradesh one, suggesting strongly that it is not variations in socio-economic background which are mainly responsible for regional differentials in child mortality and that cultural identity exerts a powerful and independent effect on the intermediate variables and through them the various mortality outcomes which result.

The main proximate variables involved in the regional differential in childhood mortality appeared to be the demographic variables of sex and parity; differences in the level of household hygiene and sanitation and in the use of preventive immunizations, both of which influence the incidence of illness; and antenatal care and the institution of delivery, which influence deaths soon after birth. Health-care in illness was not found to be an important factor, especially for the younger children, whose families theoretically had access to similar health services.

We now have a picture of regional differentials in demographic behaviour and the proximate variables through which these emerge. But what leads to these regional differentials in the intermediate variables and in these indices of demographic behaviour? We have already controlled the external physical environment (not just in terms of sanitation but also in terms of access to services) and household socio-economic circumstances.[1] In addition, we find that these demographic differentials persist even if we control for the relatively manipulable maternal characteristics of education and employment. So what remains? Our study led us to conclude that all the above variables, especially those concerned with maternal attributes, are important enough. But over and above these is something which seems less obviously amenable to outside control. This is the variable of regional or cultural background. We are inclined to agree with Cleland and Wilson (1987) who compared the European historical experience and the contemporary experience in developing countries to conclude that 'differences between cultures in terms of language, religion, customs or values may either inhibit or facilitate the adoption of family limitation or other novel forms of behaviour'. We would include the control of childhood mortality in these 'other novel forms of behaviour', so that demographic events as a whole can be viewed as being strongly influenced by cultural background.

But obviously it is not a language or geographic area itself which is progressive or conservative. These indicators of cultural identity function as a proxy for other characteristics of a population which determine their behaviour. It is a central conclusion of this book that one of the most important such characteristics which is culturally differentiated is the position of women. The 'position' or 'status' of women is a complicated and often confused concept (for a discussion of some of the complications and sources of confusion, see Mason 1984), but in the present context, that is, while examining its relation to demographic behaviour, only three separate (but interrelated) aspects of women's status were considered to be relevant:

(*a*) the extent of women's exposure to the outside world;

(*b*) the extent of women's interaction with this non-familial world; and

(*c*) the extent of female autonomy in decision-making.

While all three aspects may be considered either in absolute terms or in comparison to some other group, for example that of men, it appears that in the case of regional differentials in fertility and overall child mortality, regional differentials in the absolute levels of the above indicators of female position are sufficient to provide an explanation, once other socio-economic and environmental variables are controlled.

As for the conjectured links between women's status as defined in this way and demographic behaviour, Chapter 4 found important regional differences in three directly fertility-related variables: age at marriage, the use of modern contraception to compensate for reduced breast-feeding lengths, and the termination of childbearing. It also found corresponding regional differences in the numbers of children desired and in attitudes towards birth control. That is, final differences in marital fertility are an outcome of volition and not of differences in fecundity. It was hypothesized that with greater exposure to and interaction with the world outside the home, the women from Tamil Nadu were able not only to acquire information about the physical process of birth control, but, more importantly, to develop positive attitudes towards a smaller family size and a willingness to innovate (which is what the adoption of contraception involves) to achieve these smaller completed family sizes, even in the face of other innovations such as reduced breast-feeding, which should theoretically lead to increased fertility. In particular, female seclusion not being the norm in this culture, there was almost inevitably a much greater exposure to the forces encouraging fertility control, especially in these days of an aggressive family-planning campaign whose messages are difficult to avoid the minute one steps out of one's household in a typical urban area.

Going briefly one step back, to regional differences in the women's micro-economic situations, it is easy to see how the improved position of women (according to our present definition) increases the opportunity costs of childbearing and reduces the need for several children because of the personal and social supports which are much more readily available. For example, a woman who is willing and able to seek paid work is not only hampered by the birth of a child every two years, but in addition the absence of several children is also not such a terrible thing from the point of a security alternative in the eventuality of a husband's death or desertion.

On the other hand, the North Indian woman's relative restriction to the domestic and familial domain and her simultaneous as well as consequent restriction in decision-making works to affect the fertility-related variables in exactly the opposite way, so that higher fertility is more or less a foregone conclusion. But finally, one must add the damper that it does not necessarily follow from this that the self-perceived welfare of the Tamil women is greater. An astonishingly high proportion (over 95 per cent) of women from both regional groups maintained that they were generally happy and contented with life. Either ignorance really is bliss or we need to use much more culture-specific notions of individual welfare and aims (for a very interesting discussion of the problem of differential perception of reality including 'illusions about it' see Kynch and Sen 1983; Sen 1987).

The argument relating the position of women to levels of child mortality is more or less in the same vein as the preceding one on women's position and fertility, so it will not be repeated. The relevant elements are the greater exposure to healthier child-rearing practices, the greater willingness to accept modern medical care (but only in the area of immunizations and childbirth; for care in illness our more conservative North Indian women are as partial to the Western-style local physician), and the greater ability to practice what they learn without conflicting with other decision-makers in the household.

Earlier in this section, it was said that absolute levels of female status are the prime factors influencing demographic behaviour; the position relative to males is less relevant. To understand gender differences in physical well-being, it is now necessary to partly retract that statement. For while fertility and child mortality can be influenced purely by the absolute values of our indicators of female position, greater gender inequality in these indicators is most certainly involved in a sex ratio of child mortality in our Uttar Pradesh sample which is so adverse to girls. The absolute low levels of extra-household interaction and control on household decisions in the women from this group do not offer a good enough explanation for their daughters dying so much more easily than their sons. We need to bring in the negative association between this absolute level of female position and the extent of gender inequality in it. The predominantly male domestic and public power structure naturally leads to a devaluation of females both as adults and as children. We will not enter here into a detailed discussion of what leads to this greater gender inequality, for example, factors such as the prevailing kinship system, the low economic productivity of women, or a high non-economic physical seclusion system. But an unfortunate irony is worth mentioning. This is the fact that women are among the first to perceive their lesser economic and (often) social worth in the household and quick to internalize the norms associated with it, so that in this kind of situation, even when they do have some control over resources they think it only right to use these selectively to favour boys more than girls: witness for example the increased responsibility for a sick child's treatment for educated women in Uttar Pradesh which came out in Chapter 3 along with a simultaneous increase in the sex differential in health-care use and mortality as discussed in Chapter 6. This example forcefully brings out the need not only to improve the exposure, interaction, and autonomy status of women, but also to improve their 'perceptions' about this new reality in their lives at the same time.

The above summary along with Chapters 4, 5, and 6, while seeking a connection between women's status and demographic behaviour, have repeatedly felt the need to distinguish between two possible pathways of influence, the direct and the indirect. By the direct pathway is meant the effect of women's status on actual needs and desires—for sons and for children as a whole—resulting in effects on wanted fertility as well as on gender discrimination within the household. But, as effective in its impact was believed to be the indirect link between women's status and demographic behaviour; this link was the consequence of women's position on their ability to influence events in any direction, resulting in regional differences in fertility, child mortality, and sex differentials in physical welfare, independently of underlying preferences in these areas. Norms of female seclusion and limited economic independence for women have far-reaching effects on a woman's ability to acquire and to use information on fertility and health maintenance and, in the North Indian case, can intensify existing gender inequalities within the home. While previous chapters are littered with examples of such indirect effects, it might be useful to repeat here one example each of these indirect connections between women's status and fertility, child mortality, and sex differences in welfare: the greater North Indian gap between women who want no more children and women who currently use contraception; the greater North Indian disinclination to have a hospital-based childbirth; and the greater North Indian propensity to keep girls and women away from a male doctor.

Education is one way of raising the position of women on our demographically relevant indicators of women's status (see Caldwell 1979; Caldwell, Reddy, and Caldwell 1982; Caldwell, Reddy, and Caldwell 1983, for a discussion of the impressive range of changes pertaining to demographic behaviour possible by education). But we find that there are also intrinsic cultural differences in the position of women on these above indicators, which have their roots in something more ancient than the spread of modern education, although education certainly has a substantial impact even in groups in which women are relatively more independent to begin with. Chapter 3 documented some of the regional differences in the position of women which persisted even among the uneducated or the unemployed women. That is, the South Indian sample in our survey was found to have a history and a culture of greater freedom in movement and autonomy in household decisions than the women from northern India, which could not be explained away only by their higher rates of education and employment (indeed, these educational and employment differentials are themselves a reflection of differentials in women's position).

Instead, in Chapter 3, a case was made for considering these attributes of female status to be influenced by two aspects of the culture: marriage and kinship systems, and women's real and potential economic roles. Both these aspects were considered cultural rather than socio-economic because they were more common across different socio-economic groups within the same culture than across cultural groups within a socio-economic category. That is, although they might have their origins in economic factors, these practices are now sufficiently institutionalized not to be strongly connected with the immediate socio-economic circumstances of the individual household.

7.2. Some Policy Implications

Nowhere in the social sciences is a purely academic discussion on a topic more unwelcome than in demography.[2] One must pinpoint and discuss the policy implications of one's results if one is to be taken at all seriously. However, in fairness it must also be added that these expectations are not merely to justify the expense of a research study (and field research is admittedly a costly affair); such expectations also exist because demography is one of the subjects in which the world of theory and the world of reality are the most closely linked; we have much less of the esoteric 'if–then' kind of statements which increasingly characterize most of the other social sciences. Moreover, and more importantly, demographic behaviour is rapidly becoming that facet of human behaviour considered to be most in need of change if life is to improve for the world as a whole and for any specific part of it (in which case the direction of the needed change can vary drastically). It is also, in spite of our repeated failure, believed to be an area which is amenable to manipulation, if only we can get our basic premiss right. Fortunately this study has thrown up several policy suggestions, some very specific and others of a more general but nevertheless practical kind.

To begin with, there is the policy relevance of the central theme of this study, that demographic behaviour is a function of (among other things, of course) cultural or regional background. This means that policies to influence this behaviour cannot afford to be culture-blind. It is fine to have a centrally funded programme (as is the family-planning programme of the Government of India, for example), but the actual content of the programme needs to be made much more flexible to suit local realities.[3] It is not enough to provide standardized services or to push for economic growth, in the expectation that demographic behaviour will automatically, and soon, change in the desired direction. Institutions and norms, whatever their origins, tend to exist more along regional or cultural lines rather than socio-economic ones and, secondly, tend often to linger on long after there is no felt need for them even in those socio-economic groups which initially gave rise to them. For instance, the norms governing village exogamy may have their roots in agricultural systems which required a policy of expansion and in turn lead to norms about female seclusion and female economic activity, but village exogamy and low rates of female labour-force participation today exist in much of North India in spite of several changes in agriculture and the economy. Ignoring this hold of tradition leads to the common mistake in policy-making of treating culture as, to quote McNicoll and Cain (1990*b*), 'pervading but only marginally constraining the individual level transactions and interests that give rise to institutional patterns'. But of course culture is not a genetic or immutable concept and, to quote de Beauvoir (1974), 'one is not born, but rather becomes, a woman'. Just as culture-specific practices and attitudes have developed under certain historical conditions, in the long run one would expect a different set of attitudes and practices to become institutionalized with a change in socio-economic conditions. Economic growth is therefore certainly one important way of achieving change in women's status and in demographic behaviour. But if one is seeking more immediate effects, the findings from this book suggest that economic growth needs some non-economic help.

This kind of culture-specific approach recognizes the special status of regions of low female status for achieving fertility control. But what about health and mortality? Our results indicate that even in these areas it is not enough to specify some general norms such as one Primary Health Centre per 30 000 rural population. The health culture of the North Indian region is very different from that of South India, especially when it comes to the use of modern health services by girls and women. The consequent sex differential in child mortality has already been discussed in earlier chapters; so has the feeling that it is not necessarily discrimination against girls which is at work: the desire to protect them from the outside world in a situation of overall high female conservatism is often also an important motive for postponing the medical care of their illnesses until absolutely necessary or even until it is too late.

While the long-term strategy to combat this conservatism is literally to demolish it by improving the social and economic position of women in the directions discussed at the beginning of this chapter, our findings strongly recommend several immediate policies to improve the health of women and children, especially female children. Such measures would fall in the general category of interventions that overcome the indirect or unintentional links between women's position and demographic behaviour. Among these would be the development of good domiciliary services for antenatal care and childbirth. There is such a strong tradition of home deliveries all over the country, but especially in northern India, that this should be exploited by the health-care system; the financial savings caused by fewer hospital births can very usefully be channelled into relatively greater investments in midwives and female medical staff for North India. This is also an important step towards increasing the access of girls and women to prompt medical care in illness; the inhibitions felt about being examined by a male doctor are a significant contributor to lower health-care use for girls.

In the same vein, our study points to the need for more culture-specific services in other areas as well. Public services such as taps and toilets are less useful to the typical North Indian households, again because of the restrictions on the public movements of women. Not only are such services therefore wasteful because of underutilization, more importantly they make no impact on household sanitation and hygiene levels. For example, the water that collects because of the women's insistence on bathing (even if fully clothed) away from prying male eyes cannot but be a potential breeding ground for all kinds of disease organisms. The answer may be somewhat expensive but is still worth it in the long run: public baths (rather than taps in the open) and toilets for women need to allow for much greater privacy than is currently the case. This is a particularly important consideration for the present-day urban slum, where space and money restrictions make private facilities impossible but where, as our study illustrates, migration of women from some parts of the country has not necessarily led to an erosion of traditional fears and inhibitions. Government schools, fortunately, do cater to the conservative need for sex segregation of children and, whatever the theoretical advantages of coeducation, should continue to be so segregated if female drop-out rates are not to become even higher than they already are.

While on the importance of taking culture into account in planning, a special need of the South Indian (or any other relatively 'modern') region should be mentioned. This relates to the finding (in our study as well as in a recent all-India survey: NCAER 1985) that in groups from southern India the resort to private (that is paid) medical services is much greater than in North India. We feel that one simple practical reason which is at least partly responsible for this greater eschewal of government facilities is their inconvenient timing. As the women from South Inda are more likely to be working than those from North India and as most governmental health facilities function during the day (usually in the late morning), the working woman is forced to seek the services of the private practitioner who is available at a less unsuitable time.

On the other hand, this attempt to promote strategies for health and family planning which are sympathetic to cultural differences risks getting carried away and ignoring the culture-neutral policy implications which arise from this study. For our two regional groups did also have a lot of problems in common which are in fact common to the country as a whole. The first of these is related to the clear demonstration in Chapter 5 that when health services are easily available there is a great readiness to use them whatever the cultural background of the clients (except in the case of services for hospital deliveries and to a certain extent preventive immunizations). That is, the modern handling of an illness episode is a habit which is very easily acquired provided the services are easily available as well as compatible with certain cultural values (for example, have sufficient female staff). This question of accessibility needs to be taken into account while making pronouncements on regional differentials in rates of use. In fact, as Bose (1987) points out, the much cited example of the state of Kerala's primacy in utilizing health care services should be at least partly seen in the context of the fact that, even with the same primary health centre or sub-centre–population ratios as other states, Kerala would have a much higher physical accessibility index because of its greater density of population and a highly developed system of roads.

Then there is the question of the role of the health service in a country such as India. All confirmed critics of government programmes have pointed out the unduly high proportion of this system's time that is taken up by family-planning and curative activities. They suggest that prevention needs much more attention. Prevention seems to be equated with immunization, and to its credit the national health-care system has in recent years been trying valiantly to improve its record in this field (though not successfully enough for it to have reached the elusive UNICEF goal of universal immunization by 1990). But our data suggest that immunization is only one aspect of prevention that the health system needs to concern itself with. The dissemination of information and education on health-related matters is another equally important aspect which seems somehow to have been left by the wayside. Even with such a high level of use of health services as in our study, the women we spoke to continue to believe that colostrum is bad for a baby, that a newborn's digestive system needs to be flushed with castor oil immediately after birth, that an ill infant needs a doctor less urgently than an ill older child, or that liquid intake should be drastically reduced during a bout of diarrhoea. (But then medical opinions on these matters also change so fast, according to some of our more cynical respondents; indeed just fifty years ago we have the Wisers (Wiser and Wiser 1971) cautioning mothers that a child's dysentery is aggravated by overfeeding and that in such an illness breastmilk can even be fatal.) As Rosenzweig and Schultz (1982) have stressed with Colombian data, the public information component of health services can act as a partial substitute for the superior knowledge and skills of, for example, better educated mothers, and should reduce health and mortality differentials according to maternal characteristics. Palloni (1985) has made a similar prediction for Latin America in general: where health services are widely available, personal characteristics such as education should become less important determinants of health. Indeed, this problem of inadequate communication between the health-care system and the people is the most acute for those categories of clients who have the least access to other sources of information—the uneducated, the unemployed, and the physically secluded—all three of which adjectives are more likely to apply to the North Indian women in our sample than to their men or the men and women in the southern sample.

This brings us back to stress very forcefully the need to focus on women in any attempts to change demographic behaviour. We have already discussed the independent effect of cultural or regional background on indices of demographic behaviour. But obviously this background itself is not amenable to manipulation; what can be manipulated are some of the links in the chain between regional background and demographic behaviour, most importantly, female education and employment levels. But the mixed blessings of these two factors, at least in the initial stages, must be recorded. Our results indicate that education tends to lower fertility and child mortality, but increase the sex differential in child mortality. On the other hand, female employment tends to lower fertility and lower the sex differential in child mortality, but increase the overall level of child mortality. It also probably worsens the health of the woman herself, since the burden of housekeeping means that employment involves in effect a double shift of work. The policy implications of this are confusing, to say the least, but if we were forced to plump for one, education is probably the better alternative. It is true that the level of sex discrimination tends to go up, but absolute levels of mortality do fall for both boys and girls (see also Mosley 1983). And then, of course, there is the subsequent possibility that education will lead to employment, in which case the conservatism regarding girls or the discrimination against girls should also fall according to our hypothesis. Moreover, if such employment is an outcome of rising education rather than rising poverty, it is more likely to be of the kind where childcare does not suffer, so that perhaps overall levels of child mortality will not rise after all.

But even if education is needed more immediately to affect fertility and mortality decline, one cannot overstress the role of economic independence in raising women's status in general, greater gender equality in physical well-being being just one of the outcomes of such a rise in status.[4] As stressed so eloquently by Woolf (1929), 'What a change in temper a fixed income will bring about!' The good temper should arise out of a sense of independence as well as the knowledge that 'money dignifies what is frivolous if unpaid for'. And it is this independence which reduces the need for several children at the same time as it increases the ability to rear them well. The 'room of one's own' sought by Woolf for women is real for the aspiring woman writer; but only partly metaphorical even in the case of our less ambitious poor woman from North India. As several chapters have brought out, her access to and use of physical space are a major constraint on her ability to make a better or longer life for herself and her children, especially her girl children.

The use of the word 'herself' in the last sentence is deliberate. While this book has treated demographic behaviour largely as children being born and children dying, the real world also has adults living and adults dying. As discussed in Basu (1992), the status of women has an important bearing on the quality of life, the length of life, and the sex differentials in these two indicators among adults as well. Quite apart from quality-of-life indicators to do with the realisation of a creative or economic potential, one can think of several demographically interesting indicators of the quality of life which are affected by the position of women. One such indicator is specific to the rural–urban migration situation in the Third World today. This is the effect of women's position on the nature of the migration process. More specifically, as discussed briefly in Chapter 2, conjugal separation is an important conse-quence of migration in areas where women do not work. Or, to put it more correctly, women are more likely to migrate with men in situations where they are likely to join the labour-force in the city, whether the reasons for this concern the job opportunites available or their ówn inhibitions about making use of these opportunities. This is one of the reasons why several studies (see, for instance, Chapter 2 above; Singh 1984; Banerjee 1984) have found a much higher masculinity among migrant populations from North India than among those from the South, whatever the town or city of destination.

Finally, a word about our motivations. Throughout this section we have had the underlying assumption that the ultimate goals are reduced fertility and mortality. While this is not really the place to enter a discussion on the justification of these goals regarding fertility (reducing mortality justifies itself), we feel that Table 7.1 should be presented as well. Happiness is an amorphous concept it is true, but perhaps one ought not to dismiss too rudely the finding that for both regional groups, there was this consistent relationship between numbers of living children and general contentment with life.

7.3. Discussion

We would like to begin this last section of the book by pointing out that in our zeal to demonstrate cultural differences in the status of women and, correspondingly, in demographic behaviour, we have neglected to add that the South Indian advantage is still only relative. That is, on absolute levels, even this region has a long way to go and it is somewhat dismaying to find that there is a (fortunately small) tendency for our Tamil migrants sometimes to be worse off in this respect, especially on the matter of stated gender equality, than their counterparts in the home state. That is, the North Indian culture is able to overwhelm some of the more

Table 7.1. Women's self-perceived happiness according to
their number of living children

Region and number of children	% of women who are happy with life		
	Age-group		
	< 30	30–49	All ages
Uttar Pradesh			
0	76	38	71
1–3	88	87	88
4 +	92	90	91
Tamil Nadu			
0	92	50	84
1–3	94	89	92
4 +	93	95	95

progressive attributes of the southern one. Thus we have the
phenomenon of only 50 per cent of the Tamil women feeling that
sons and daughters need to be equally educated; the comparable
figure for Uttar Pradesh being 57 per cent. Similarly, about 8 per
cent of the South Indian women felt that boys deserve better food
than girls, compared to a figure of 3 per cent for Uttar Pradesh.
Fortunately, these values do not seem to have become internalized
enough to affect behaviour, so that we still find that in 13 per
cent of North Indian households the men eat meat, and the
women do not, while this percentage is close to zero in Tamil
Nadu. Similar sex differentials are seen in meat consumption by
children. However, it must be added that these sex differences in
consumption are symbolic rather than real; that is, they do not
really lead to overall nutritional discriminition against females
(see Chapter 6 above, and O'Laughlin 1974, for a fuller discussion
of this point); what they do is reinforce the perceived overall lesser
importance of women and girls.

Next, how far are our findings generalizable to Tamil Nadu and
Uttar Pradesh in particular and North and South India as a whole?
After all, in the interest of controlling the environment, we have
had to resort to studying migrant groups. The standard objections
to this are that such groups are unrepresentative because, firstly,
they must belong to an especially innovative group to have made
the decision to migrate in the first place, and secondly, they must

have adopted some of the behavioural and attitudinal patterns of the new city. Our answers to these objections are that while they are indeed valid, their impact is mitigated greatly because the great majority of these are first-generation migrants and therefore have not had much time to assimilate the local culture, and the primary respondents in the survey were the ever-married women, who have mainly reached the capital city either while accompanying their husbands or as new brides when the single males among the migrants went home to marry. That is, they have not been the decision-makers in the act of moving out of their home states and therefore there is little reason to expect them to have been particularly innovative or liberated to begin with.

Moreover, the migration history of our two groups of women is remarkably similar. For both groups the mean age at which the women came to Delhi is 19 years and the mean number of years since arrival is 12 for the Uttar Pradesh women and 13 for the Tamil women. Therefore, any changes in attitudes and behaviour that have occurred with migration will, according to our hypothesis, again reflect cultural differences in the willingness to innovate. Indeed, this is the right time to quote Lesthaeghe's (1983) remark about the demographic transition in Europe and apply it to our sample: 'while many aspects of behaviour changed during the demographic transition, the relative openness of regions to new ideas often remained remarkably stable'. Our data also suggest similar regional predispositions, because of which cultural differences in demographic behaviour persist even after we control for the effects of the environment, household socio-economic status, and also such variables of women's status as education and employment.

Finally, how many of our findings can be generalized to include other cultures and geographic areas? This field study should be treated as illustrative rather than specific, in that the central results are applicable to a wide range of cultures and geographic areas, most strongly within South Asia and, less strongly but still significantly, to other developing areas as well. This is because the links that were found between women's status and demographic behaviour conceivably exist to a lesser or greater degree in any population group. Wherever women are unable to interact freely with the outside world, their sources of information are limited as is their ability to act on any information obtained. Similarly, whenever women are economically active, their control over their own lives as well as the lives of their families can be expected to increase, however marginally, and, less palatably, their physical ability to exercise such control may simultaneously actually decrease, as is seen, for example, in the possible negative impact of women's employment on child mortality as discussed in Chapter 5.

The role of economic independence for women has been stressed throughout this book as one of the major routes to reduced fertility and greater gender equality within the household (see also Mitra 1978). And on both these counts, the North India–South India comparison is not an isolated example. As several writers have pointed out (see, in particular, Boserup 1970), the North Indian pattern of female seclusion and low economic activity is part of a wider region that includes Pakistan and the Middle Eastern Arab countries, while the South India pattern has its parallels in South East Asia (see also Caldwell 1986). In turn, it is interesting that from a survey of 46 peasant communities around the world, Michaelson and Goldschmidt (1971) concluded that in five of the six societies in which women did much of the agricultural labour, there was no clear evidence of male dominance. And of the 37 in which the female contribution to agriculture was relatively small, male dominance was strong in 34.

At the same time it needs to be admitted that female autonomy as proxied by economic roles may be illusory. Nothing illustrates this better than the situation of women in tropical Africa. As Caldwell and Caldwell (1985) point out with the Yoruba example, reproductive decisions and family economics are largely separated here. In spite of the unique economic independence of Yoruba women, they continue to see reproduction as a religious obligation to their husbands' lineage and children as the primary source of social and psychological security in a system of pervasive polygyny. But these are also cultural rather than socio-economic motivations for high fertility and, in a sense, they are analogous to the son preference (which is largely absent in Africa) that pervades South Asian society. The African example therefore fits more neatly into our model of culture and women's status on the one hand and demographic behaviour on the other, if traditional religion and the system of polygyny rather than generalized autonomy are the intervening variables. In such a situation the more relevant fertility-reducing agent related to women's status is probably the modernization that comes with education rather than the self-sufficiency that comes with economic independence.

Patriarchal kinship systems are but one way of limiting the options open to women. One can think of other ways which are, fortunately, more amenable to change and which may even overcome the disadvantages of patriarchy: economic opportunity structures, the access to education and information, the level of physical and social security, and the extra-familial cushions against debility and disaster. All these exist in different ways in different settings and potentially affect women's position on the indicators described in Chapter 3 and, as a result, on expressed demographic behaviour. As much research has concluded, there certainly seems to be a plausible case for relating historical population changes at least partly to changes in women's roles. Given the seemingly unconnected range of socio-economic conditions and demographic regimes that exist in the contemporary developing world, it would appear that there is an even stronger case to be made for including the position of women in any realistic explanation of demographic behaviour today.

NOTES

1. The range of incomes covered in the study sample was very small, so income was not likely to have been a confounding factor in the findings. Moreover, within this narrow range of incomes, no clear relations were found between income and fertility and child survival.
2. But this, as Demeny (1988) has pointed out, was not always so; as late as 1959, the US National Science Foundation Survey, *The Study of Population*, referred in its introduction to those who sought a policy role for demographers as 'fringe groups'.
3. This is recognized (at least on paper) and officially the family-planning programme is supposed to function differentially (that is, more intensely) in the Northern or Hindi-speaking belt of the country.
4. This is not to suggest that women who are not visibly employed have no economic value to the household. As several studies on the time allocation of poor women have pointed out, even the contribution of unemployed women to the household economy can be significant and indispensable. But as long as there is no perception of such contribu-

tion, it is possible for there not to develop a rationale for greater equality in the quality of life of the two sexes. One wishful alternative to changing the economic roles of women may therefore lie in educating them (and, even more importantly, other household members including the men) to have a better appreciation of women's economic worth, even when they are not employed in the conventional sense.

References

AABY, P. (1988), *Malnourished or Overinfected: An Analysis of the Determinants of Acute Measles Mortality*, Copenhagen: Copenhagen University.

ALAM, I. and CLELAND, J. (1981), 'Illustrative Analysis: Recent Fertility Trends in Sri Lanka', *World Fertility Survey Scientific Reports*, no. 25.

ALLAND, A. (1970), *Adaptation in Cultural Evolution: An Approach to Medical Anthropology*, New York: Columbia University Press.

ANDERSON, B. A. (1986), 'Regional and Cultural Factors in the Decline of Marital Fertility in Western Europe', in Coale and Watkins (eds.) *Decline of Fertility*.

APPADURAI, A. (1981), 'Gastropolitics in Hindu South Asia', *American Ethnologist*, vol.18, no. 3.

ARNOLD, F. (1987), 'The Effect of Sex Preference on Fertility and Family Planning: Empirical Evidence', *Population Bulletin of the United Nations*, nos. 23/24.

ARNOLD, F. and ZHAOXIANG, L. (1986), 'Sex Preference, Fertility and Family Planning in China', *Population and Development Review*, vol. 12, no. 2.

ARORA, Y. L., PRAKASAN, C. P. and KARKAL, M. (1979), 'Infant Mortality and its Correlates in Greater Bombay', *Health and Population—Perspectives and Issues*, vol. 2, no. 4.

ARRIAGA, E. (1980), 'Direct Estimates of Infant Mortality Differentials from Birth Histories', *Proceedings of the World Fertility Survey Conference, London*, Geneva: International Statistical Institute.

AZIZ, K. M. A. (1977), 'Present Trends in Medical Consultation prior to Death in Rural Bangladesh', *Bangladesh Medical Journal*, vol. 6, no. 53.

BANERJEE, B. (1984), 'Rural to Urban Migration and Conjugal Separation: An Indian Case Study', *Economic Development and Cultural Change*, vol. 32, no. 4.

BANERJEE, D. (1973), 'Health Behaviour of Rural Populations: Impact of Rural Health Services', *Economic and Political Weekly*, vol. 8, no. 51.

BARDHAN, P. K. (1974), 'On Life and Death Questions', *Economic and Political Weekly*, vol. 19, nos. 32–4.

BASU, A. M. (1985), 'Family Planning and the Emergency: An Unanticipated Consequence', *Economic and Political Weekly*, vol. 20, no. 10.

—— (1987) 'Household Influences on Childhood Mortality: The Evidence from Historical and Recent Mortality Trends', *Social Biology*, vol. 34, nos. 3–4.

____ (1989), 'Is Discrimination in Food really Necessary for Explaining Sex Differentials in Childhood Mortality?', *Population Studies*, vol. 43, no. 2.

____ (1990), 'Cultural Influences on Child Health in a Delhi Slum: And in What Way is Urban Poverty Preferable to Rural Poverty?', in J. C. Caldwell and G. Santow (eds.), *Cultural, Social and Behavioural Determinants of Health: What is the Evidence?* Canberra: Australian National University.

____ (1992), 'The Status of Women and the Quality of Life among the Poor', *Cambridge Journal of Economics* (forthcoming).

____ (forthcoming), 'Cultural Influences on the Timing of First Births in India', *Population Studies*.

____ and SUNDAR, R. (1988), 'The Domestic Servant as Family Planning Innovator: An Indian Case Study', *Studies in Family Planning*, vol. 19, no. 5.

____ BASU, K. and RAY, R. (1987), 'Migrants and the Native Bond: An Analysis of Micro Level Data from Delhi', *Economic and Political Weekly*, annual number, vol. 22.

____ and BASU, K. (1991), 'Women's Economic Roles and Child Survival; Illustrated with the Case of India', *Health Transition Review*, vol. 1, no. 1.

BASU, K., JONES E. L. and SCHLICHT, E. (1987), 'The Growth and Decay of Custom: The Role of the New Institutional Economics in Economic History', *Explorations in Economic History*, vol. 24, no. 1.

BEAN, L. L., MINEAU, G. P. and ANDERTON D. L. (1990), *Fertility Change on the American Frontier*, Berkeley: University of California Press.

BHATIA, J. (1978) 'Ideal Number and Sex Composition of Children in India', *Journal of Family Welfare*, vol. 24, no. 4. •

BLACK, R. E. (1984), 'Diarrhoeal Diseases and Child Morbidity and Mortality', *Population and Development Review*, supplement to vol. 10.

BLEEK, W. (1987), 'Lying Informants: A Fieldwork Experience from Ghana', *Population and Development Review*, vol. 13, no. 2.

BLOOM, D. E. and REDDY, P. H. (1984), *Age Patterns of Women at Marriage, Cohabitation and First Birth in India*, Center for Population Studies, Harvard University, discussion paper 84–6.

BONGAARTS, J. (1978), 'A Framework for Analyzing the Proximate Determinants of Fertility', *Population and Development Review*, vol. 4, no. 1.

____ (1982), 'The Fertility Inhibiting Effects of the Intermediate Fertility Variables', *Studies in Family Planning*, vol. 13, nos. 6–7.

____ (1983), 'The Proximate Determinants of Natural Marital Fertility', in Bulatao and Lee (eds.), *Determinants of Fertility*.

____ (1987), 'Does Family Planning Reduce Infant Mortality Rates?', *Population and Development Review*, vol. 13, no. 2.

_____ and POTTER, R. G. (1979), 'The Fertility Effect of Seasonal Migration and Seasonal Variation in Fecundability: "Test of a Useful Approximation under more General Conditions" ', *Demography*, vol. 16, no. 3.

_____ (1983), *Fertility, Biology and Behavior: An Analysis of the Proximate Determinants*, New York: Academic Press.

BOSE, A. (1987), *For Whom the Target Tolls: A Critique of Family Planning Incentives, Cash Awards and Targets*, presidential address to the 12th annual conference of the Indian Association for the Study of Population, Allahabad, India.

_____ (1988), *In Search of a New Strategy for Family Planning in India*, presidential address to the 13th annual conference of the Indian Association for the Study of Population, Waltair, India.

BOSERUP, E. (1970), *Women's Role in Economic Development*, New York: St. Martin's Press.

BRASS, W. (1978), 'Screening Procedures for Detecting Errors in Maternity History Data', World Fertility Survey Technical Paper 810, London.

BULATAO, R. A. and LEE, R. D. (eds.) (1983), *Determinants of Fertility in Developing Countries*, New York: Academic Press.

CAIN, M. (1982), 'Perspectives on Family and Fertility in Developing Countries', *Population Studies*, vol. 26, no. 2.

_____ (1984), *Women's Status and Fertility in Developing Countries: Son Preference and Economic Security*, World Bank Staff Working Papers, no. 682.

_____ (1985), 'On the Relationship between Landholding and Fertility', *Population Studies*, vol. 39, no. 1.

CALDWELL, J. C. (1979), 'Education as a Factor in Mortality Decline', *Population Studies*, vol. 33, no. 3.

_____ (1981), 'Influence of Maternal Education on Infant and Child Mortality', *Proceedings of the International Union for the Scientific Study of Population Conference, Manila*.

_____ (1986), 'Routes to Low Mortality in Poor Countries', *Population and Development Review*, vol. 12, no. 2.

_____ and CALDWELL, P. (1985), *Cultural Forces Tending to Sustain High Fertility in Tropical Africa*, PHN Technical Note 85–16, Canberra, Australian: National University.

_____ , REDDY, P. H. and CALDWELL, P. (1982), 'The Causes of Demographic Change in Rural South India: A Micro Approach', *Population and Development Review*, vol. 8, no. 4.

_____ (1983), 'The Social Component of Mortality Decline: An Investigation in South India Employing Alternative Methodologies, *Population Studies*, vol. 37, no. 2.

CARLSSON, G. (1966), 'The Decline of Fertility: Innovation or Adjustment Process', *Population Studies*, vol. 20, no. 2.

CHAKRAVARTI, A. K. (1982), 'Diet and Disease: Some Cultural Aspects of Food Use in India', in A.G. Noble and A.K. Dutt (eds.), *India: Cultural Patterns and Processes*, Boulder, Colo.: Westview Press.

CHAUDHURY, R. H. (1982), 'The Effect of Mother's Work on Child Care, Dietary Intake and Dietary Adequacy of Pre-School Children', *Bangladesh Development Studies*, vol. 10, no. 4.

—— (1984), 'Determinants of Dietary Intake and Dietary Adequacy for Pre-School Children in Bangladesh', *Food and Nutrition Bulletin*, vol. 6, no. 4.

—— (1987), 'Dietary Adequacy and Sex Bias: Pre-School Children in Rural Bangladesh', *Social Action*, vol. 37, no. 2.

CHEN, L. C. (1982), 'Where have the Women Gone? Insights from Bangladesh on the Low Sex Ratios of India's Population', *Economic and Political Weekly*, vol. 17, no. 10.

—— (1983), 'Child Survival: Levels, Trends and Determinants', in Bulatao, and Lee (eds.) *Determinants of Fertility*.

—— HUQ, E. and D'SOUZA, S. (1981), 'Sex Bias in the Family Allocation of Food and Health Care in Rural Bangladesh', *Population and Development Review*, vol. 7, no. 1.

—— RAHMAN, A. and SARDAR, J. (1980), 'Epidemiology and Causes of Death among Children in a Rural Area of Bangladesh', *International Journal of Epidemiology*, vol. 9.

—— CHOWDHURY, A. K. M. A. and HUFFMAN, S. L. (1980), 'Anthropometric Assessment of Energy-Protein Malnutrition and Subsequent Risk of Mortality among Pre-School Aged Children', *The American Journal of Clinical Nutrition*, vol. 33, pp. 1836–45.

—— AHMED, S., GESCHE, M. and MOSLEY, W. H. (1974), 'A Prospective Study of Birth Interval Dynamics in Rural Bangladesh', *Population Studies*, vol. 28, no. 2.

CHIDAMBARAM, V. C. and ZODEGEKAR, A.V. (1969), 'Increasing Female Age at Marriage in India and its Impact on the First Birth Interval: An Empirical Analysis', *Proceedings of the IUSSP Conference London*, Liège, Belgium: International Union for the Scientific Study of Population.

CHUTIKUL, S. (1986), 'Malnourished Children: An Economic Approach to the Causes and Consequences in Rural Thailand', papers of the East–West Population Institute, no. 102.

CLELAND, J. (1985), 'Marital Fertility Decline in Developing Countries', in Cleland and Hobcraft (eds.) *Reproductive Change*.

—— and HOBCRAFT J. N. (eds.) (1985), *Reproductive Change in Developing Countries: Insights from the World Fertility Survey*, Oxford: Oxford University Press.

—— and WILSON, C. (1987), 'Demand Theories of the Fertility Transition: An Iconoclastic View', *Population Studies*, vol. 41, no. 1.

—— VERRALL, J. and VAESSEN, M. (1983), 'Preferences for the Sex of Children and their Influence on Reproductive Behaviour', World Fertility Survey Comparative Studies, Cross-national summaries, no. 27.

COALE, A. J. (1973), *The Demographic Transition*, Liège, International Union for the Scientific Study of Population.

—— (1991), *Some Relations among Cultural Traditions, Nuptiality and Fertility*, Office of Population Research, Princeton, NJ, mimeo.

—— and TYE, C. Y. (1961), 'The Significance of Age Patterns in High Fertility Populations', *Milbank Memorial Fund Quarterly*, vol. 39, no. 4.

—— and WATKINS, S. C. (eds.) (1986), *The Decline of Fertility in Europe*, Princeton, NJ: Princeton University Press.

COCHRANE, S. (1979), 'Fertility and Education: What do we Really Know?', World Bank Staff Occasional Paper, no. 26.

CRAFTS, N. F. R. (1989), 'Duration of Marriage, Fertility and Women's Employment Opportunities in England and Wales in 1911', *Population Studies*, vol. 43, no. 2.

DAS GUPTA, M. (1987), 'Selective Discrimination against Female Children in India', *Population and Development Review*, vol. 13, no. 1.

DAVID, P. A. and SANDERSON, W. C. (1987), 'The Emergence of a Two-Child Norm among American Birth-Controllers', *Population and Development Review*, vol. 13, no. 1.

DAVIS, K. and BLAKE, J. (1956), 'Social Structure and Fertility: An Analytical Framework', *Economic Development and Cultural Change*, vol. 9, no. 4.

DE BEAUVIOR, S. (1974), *The Second Sex*, New York: Vintage Books.

DEMENY, P. (1988), 'Social Science and Population Policy', *Population and Development Review*, vol. 14, no. 3.

Department of Health and Family Welfare (1985), *Health Statistics of India*, New Delhi: Government of India.

DE SOUZA, A. (ed.) (1978), *The Indian City: Poverty, Ecology and Urban Development*, New Delhi: Manohar Publishers.

DIXON, R. B. (1971), 'Explaining Cross-Cultural Variations in Age at Marriage and Proportions Never Marrying', *Population Studies*, vol. 25, no. 2.

DRÈZE, J. (1990), *Widows in Rural India*, London School of Economics, Development Economics Research Programme, paper no. 26, London.

—— and SEN, A. (1990), *Hunger and Public Action*, Oxford: Oxford University Press.

DRIVER, E. D. (1963), *Differential Fertility in Central India*, Princeton, NJ: Princeton University Press.

D'SOUZA, S. and CHEN, L. C. (1980), 'Sex Differentials in Mortality in Rural Bangladesh', *Population and Development Review*, vol. 6, no. 2.

DWYER, D. and BRUCE, J. (eds.) (1988), *A Home Divided: Women and Income in the Third World*, Stanford, Calf.: Stanford University Press.

DYSON, T. (1984), 'Excess Male Mortality in India', *Economic and Political Weekly*, vol. 19, no. 10.

―――― (1988), 'Excess Female Mortality in India: Uncertain Evidence on a Narrowing Differential' in K. Srinivasan and S. Mukherji (eds.), *Dynamics of Population and Family Welfare*, Bombay: Himalaya Publishing House.

―――― (1989), 'A Further Note on Trends in the Sex Differential in Mortality in India', paper presented at the IUSSP general conference of the International Union for the Scientific Study of Population, New Delhi.

―――― and MOORE, M. (1983), 'On Kinship Structure, Female Autonomy and Demographic Behaviour in India', *Population and Development Review*, vol. 9, no. 1.

EL-BADRY, M. A. (1969), 'Higher Female than Male Mortality in some Countries of South Asia: A Digest', *American Statistical Association Journal*, vol. 64, no. 3.

ERASMUS, C. J. (1961), *Man Takes Control*, Minneapolis, Minn.: University of Minnesota Press.

GARDNER, J. and MAIER, J. (1985), *Gilgamesh*, New York: Vintage Books.

GASTARDO-CONACO, C., RAMOS-JIMENEZ, P., and BARNIEGO, R. N. (1986), *Ethnicity and Fertility in the Philippines*, research notes and discussion paper, no. 54, Institute of Southeast Asian Studies, Singapore.

GIBRIL, M. A. (1979), *Evaluating Census Response Errors: A Case Study for the Gambia*, Paris: OECD.

GILLE, H. (1985), 'Policy implications', in Cleland and Hobcraft (eds.) *Reproductive Change*.

GOPALAN, C. (1987), 'Gender Bias in Health and Nutrition Care', *Nutrition Foundation of India Bulletin*, vol. 2, no. 4.

―――― and VIJAYA RAGHAVAN, K. (1969), *Nutrition Atlas of India*, Hyderabad: National Institute of Nutrition.

―――― BALASUBRAMANIUM, S., SASTRI, R. B., and RAO, K. V. (1969), *Diet Atlas of India*, Hyderabad: National Institute of Nutrition.

GRAFF, H. I. (1979), 'Literacy, Education and Fertility, Past and Present: A Critical Review', *Population and Development Review*, vol. 5, no. 1.

GREER, G. (1984), *Sex and Destiny: The Politics of Human Fertility*, New York: Harper and Row.

GULATI, S. C. (1987), 'Some Reflections on Son Preference and its Influence on Additional Desired Fertility', *Demography India*, vol. 16, no. 2.

GUNASEKARAN, S. (1988), 'Correlates of Infant Mortality in Madurai District of Tamil Nadu', in Jain and Visaria (eds.), *Infant Mortality*.

GUPTA, S. C. (1985), 'Sex Preference and Protein-Calorie Malnutrition', *The Journal of Family Welfare*, vol. 32, no. 3.

HAINES, M. R. (1989), 'Social Class Differentials during Fertility Decline: England and Wales Revisited', *Population Studies*, vol. 43, no. 2.

HALSTED, S. B., WALSH, J. A. and WARREN, K. S. (eds.) (1985), *Good Health at Low Cost*, New York: Rockefeller Foundation.

HARRIS, B. (1990), 'The Intrafamily Distribution of Hunger in South Asia', in Drèze and Sen (eds.), *Political Economy of Hunger*.

HILDERBRAND, K., HILL, A. G., RANDALL, S. and VAN DEN EERENBEEMT, M. L. (1985), 'Child Mortality and Care of Children in Rural Mali' in A.G. Hill (ed.), *Population, Health and Nutrition in the Sahel: Issues in the Welfare of Selected West African Communities*, London: Routledge and Kegan Paul.

HOBCRAFT, J. N. (1985), 'Family Building Patterns', in Cleland and Hobcraft (eds.), *Reproductive Change*.

—— McDONALD, J. and RUTSTEIN, S. O. (1983), 'Child-Spacing Effects on Infant and Early Child Mortality', *Population Index*, vol. 49, no. 4.

—— (1985), 'Demographic Determinants of Infant and Early Child Mortality: A Comparative Analysis', *Population Studies*, vol. 39, no. 3.

HUFFMAN, S. L., CHOWDHURY, A. K. M. A., CHAKRABORTY, J. and SIMPSON, N. K. (1980), 'Breast-feeding Patterns in Rural Bangladesh', *American Journal of Clinical Nutrition*, vol. 33, no. 14.

JAIN, A. K. (1985), 'Determinants of Regional Variations in Infant Mortality in Rural India', *Population Studies*, vol. 39, no. 3.

—— and BONGAARTS, J. (1981), 'Breastfeeding: Patterns, Correlates and Fertility Effects', *Studies in Family Planning*, vol. 12, no. 3.

—— and VISARIA, P. (eds.) (1988), *Infant Mortality in India: Differentials and Determinants*, New Delhi: Sage Publications.

JEFFERY, P., JEFFERY, R. and LYON, A. (1989), *Labour Pains and Labour Power: Women and Childbearing in India*, London: Zed Books.

JEJEEBHOY, S. (1981), 'Status of Women and Fertility: A Socio-Cultural Analysis of Regional Variations in Fertility in India', in K. Srinivasan and S. Mukherji (eds.), *Dynamics of Population and Family Welfare 1981*, Bombay: Himalaya Publishing House.

KANITKAR, T. and MURTHY, B. N. (1983), 'Factors Associated with Contraception in Bihar and Rajasthan: Findings from Recent Sample Surveys, in K. Srinivasan and S. Mukerji (eds.), *Dynamics of Population and Family Welfare 1983*, Bombay: Himalaya Publishing House.

KARVE, I. (1965), *Kinship Organization in India*, Bombay: Asia Publishing House.

KATONA-APTE, J. (1978), 'Urbanization, Income and Socio-Cultural Factors Relevant to Nutrition in Tamil Nadu', in de Souza (ed.), *The Indian City*.

KHAN, M. E. (1988), 'Infant Mortality in Uttar Pradesh: A Micro-Level Study', in Jain and Visaria (eds.), *Infant Mortality in India*.

____ and GUPTA, R. B. (1987), 'Familial Values, Contraception and Utilization of MCH Services in Rural Uttar Pradesh', in M. E. Khan, R. B. Gupta, C.V.S. Prasad and S.K. Ghosh Dastidar (eds.), *Performance of Family Planning in India: Observations from Bihar, Uttar Pradesh, Rajasthan and Madhya Pradesh*, Delhi: Himalaya Publishing House.

____ and PRASAD, C. V. S. (1983), *Family Planning Practices in India: Second All India Survey*, Baroda: Operations Research Group.

____ , ANKER, R., GHOSH DASTIDAR, S. K. and BHARATHI, S. (1988), 'Inequalities between Men and Women in Nutrition and Family Welfare Services', *Social Action*, vol. 38, no. 2.

KIELMANN, A. A. and Associates (1983), *Child and Maternal Health Services in Rural India: The Narangwal Experiment*, Baltimore and London: Johns Hopkins University Press.

KNODEL, J. and VAN DE WALLE, E. (1986), 'Lessons from the Past: Policy Implications of Historical Fertility Studies', in Coale and Watkins (eds.), *The Decline of Fertility*.

KOENIG, M. A. and D'SOUZA, S. (1986), 'Sex Differences in Childhood Mortality in Rural Bangladesh', *Social Science and Medicine*, vol. 22, no. 1.

KUMAR, S. (1977), 'Role of the Household Economy in Determining Child Nutrition at Low Income Levels: A Case Study of Kerala', occasional paper no. 95, Department of Agricultural Economics, Cornell University, Ithaca, NY.

KYNCH, J. and SEN, A. (1983), 'Indian Women: Well Being and Survival', *Cambridge Journal of Economics*, vol. 7, nos. 3–4.

LANGFORD, C. M. (1984), 'Sex Differentials in Mortality in Sri Lanka: Changes since the 1920s', *Journal of Biosocial Science*, vol. 16, no. 3.

LESLIE, J. and PAOLISSO, M. (eds.) (1989), *Women, Work and Child Welfare in the Third World*, Boulder, Colo.: Westview Press.

LESTHAEGHE, R. J. (1977), *The Decline of Belgian Fertility, 1800–1970*, Princeton, NJ: Princeton University Press.

____ (1983), 'A Century of Demographic and Cultural Change in Western Europe: An Exploration of Underlying Dimensions', *Population and Development Review*, vol. 9, no. 3.

LEVINSON, F. J. (1972), *Morinda: An Economic Analysis of Malnutrition Among Young Children in Rural India*, Ithaca, NY: Cornell University Press.

LIEBAN, R. W. (1977), 'The Field of Medical Anthropology', in D. Landy (ed.), *Culture, Disease and Healing: Studies in Medical Anthropology*, New York: Macmillan.

LIGHTBOURNE, R. E. and MACDONALD, A. L. (1982), *Family Size Preferences*, World Fertility Survey Comparative Studies, no. 14.

LINDENBAUM, S. (1985), *The Influence of Maternal Education on Infant and*

Child Mortality in Bangladesh, Bangladesh: International Centre for Diarrhoeal Disease Research.

LIPTON, M. (1983), *Poverty, Undernutrition and Hunger*, World Bank Staff Working Papers, no. 597, Washington, DC.

LIVI-BACCI, M. (1971), *A Century of Portuguese Fertility*, Princeton, NJ: Princeton University Press.

LODGE, D. (1984), *Small World*, London: Martin Secker and Warburg.

McDONALD, P. (1984), *Nuptiality and Completed Fertility: A Study of Starting, Stopping and Spacing Behavior*, World Fertility Survey Comparative Studies, no. 35.

____ (1985), 'Social Organization and Nuptiality in Developing Countries', in Cleland and Hobcraft (eds.), *Reproductive Change*.

McNICOLL, G. and CAIN, M. (eds.) (1990*a*), *Rural Development and Population: Institutions and Policy*, New York: Oxford University Press.

____ (1990*b*) 'Institutional Effects on Rural Economic and Demographic Change', in McNicoll and Cain (eds.), *Rural Development*.

MADAN, T. N. (1965), *Family and Kinship: A Study of the Pandits of Rural Kashmir*, Bombay: Asia Publishing House.

MANDELBAUM, D. G. (1988*a*), 'Sex Roles and Gender Relations in North India', *Economic and Political Weekly*, vol. 23, no. 10.

____ (1988*b*), *Women's Seclusion and Men's Honour*, Tucson: University of Arizona Press.

MASON, K. O. (1984), *The Status of Women: A Review of its Relationships to Fertility and Mortality*, New York: The Rockefeller Foundation.

____ and TAJ, A.M. (1987), 'Differences between Women's and Men's Reproductive Goals in Developing Countries', *Population and Development Review*, vol. 13, no. 4.

MAY, D. A. and HEER, D. M. (1968), 'Son Survivorship Motivation and Family Size in India: A Computer Simulation', *Population Studies*, vol. 22, no. 2.

MAZUMDAR, P. S. and MAZUMDAR, I. (1976), *Rural Migrants in an Urban Setting*, Delhi: Hindustan Publishing Corporation.

MENCHER, J. P. (1978), *Agriculture and Social Structure in Tamil Nadu*, New Delhi, Allied Publishers.

____ (1988), 'Women's Work and Poverty: Women's Contribution to Household Maintenance in South India', in Dwyer and Bruce (eds.), *A Home Divided*.

____ (1989), 'Women Agricultural Labourers and Land Owners in Kerala and Tamil Nadu: Some questions about Gender and Autonomy in the Household', in M. Krishnaraj and K. Chanana (eds.) *Gender and the Household Domain: Social and Cultural Dimensions*, New Delhi: Sage.

MENKEN, J. (1979), 'Seasonal Migration and Seasonal Variation in

Fecundability: Effects on Birth Rates and Birth Intervals', *Demography*, vol. 16, no. 1.

MICHAELSON, E. J. and GOLDSCHMIDT, W. (1971), 'Female Roles and Male Dominance among Peasants', *Southwestern Journal of Anthropology*, vol. 27, no. 4.

MILLER, B. D. (1981), *The Endangered Sex: Neglect of Female Children in Rural North India*, Ithaca, NY and London: Cornell University Press.

MILLER, J. (1989), 'Is the Relationship between Birth Intervals and Perinatal Mortality Spurious?', *Population Studies*, vol. 43, no. 3.

Ministry of Health and Family Welfare (1988), *Department of Family Welfare, Annual Yearbook*, New Delhi, Government of India.

MITRA, A. (1978), *India's Population: Aspects of Quality and Control*, New Delhi: Family Planning Foundation.

MOSLEY, W. H. (1983), 'Will Primary Health Care Reduce Infant and Child Mortality? A Critique of some Current Strategies with Special Reference to Africa and Asia', *IUSSP Seminar* on *Social Policy, Health Policy and Mortality Prospects, Paris*, Liège, Belgium: International Union for the Scientific Study of Population.

—— (1984), 'Child Survival: Research and Policy', *Population and Development Review*, supplement to vol. 10.

—— (1985), 'Biological and Socio-Economic Determinants of Child Survival: A Proximate Determinants Framework Integrating Fertility and Mortality Variables', *Proceedings of the IUSSP Conference, Florence*, Liège, Belgium: International Union for the Scientific Study of Population.

—— and CHEN, L. C. (1984), 'An Analytical Framework for the Study of Child Survival in Developing Countries', *Population and Development Review*, supplement to vol. 10.

NAG, M. (1980), 'How Modernization can also Increase Fertility', *Current Anthropology*, vol. 21, no. 5.

—— (1983), 'The Impact of Social and Economic Development on Mortality: A Comparative Study of Kerala and West Bengal', *Economic and Political Weekly*, annual number, vol. 18, nos. 19–21.

National Academy of Sciences (1989), *Contraception and Reproduction: Health Consequences for Women and Children in the Developing World*, Washington, DC: National Academy Press.

National Council of Applied Economic Research (1985), *Household Expenditure on Medicines and Health Care*, New Delhi: NCAER.

National Institute of Nutrition (1984), *National Nutrition Monitoring Bureau Report for the Year 1981*, Hyderabad: National Institute of Nutrition.

Nutrition Foundation of India (1988), *Profiles of Undernutrition and Underdevelopment*, NFI Scientific Report, no. 8, Delhi.

ODDY, D. J. (1970), 'Working Class Diets in Late Nineteenth Century Britain', *Economic History Review*, vol. 23, no. 2.

O'LAUGHLIN, B. (1974), 'Mediation of Contradiction: Why Mbum Women do not Eat Chicken', in M.Z. Rosaldo and L. Lamphere (eds.), *Women, Culture and Society*, Stanford, Calif.: Stanford University Press.

PALLONI, A. (1985), 'Health Conditions in Latin America and Policies for Mortality Change', in J. Vallin and A.D. Lopez (eds.), *Health Policy, Population Policy and Mortality Prospects*, Liège: Ordina Publications.

—— (1989), 'Effects of Inter-Birth Intervals on Infant and Early Childhood Mortality', in L. Ruzicka, G. Wunsch, and P. Kane (eds.), *Differential Mortality: Methodological Issues and Biosocial Factors*, Oxford: Clarendon Press.

PANIKAR, P. G. K. and SOMAN, C. R. (1984), *Health Status of Kerala: The Paradox of Economic Backwardness and Health Development*, Trivandrum, India: Centre for Development Studies.

PETTIGREW, J. (1986), 'Child Neglect in Rural Punjabi Families', *Journal of Comparative Family Studies*, vol. 17, no. 1.

POPKIN, B. N. and SOLON, F. S. (1976), 'Income, Time, the Working Mother and Child Nutriture', *Environmental Child Health*.

PREMI, M. K. (1991), 'The Growing Imbalance in India's Male–Female Ratio', *Economic Times*, New Delhi, 18 April.

PRESTON, S. H. (1985), 'Mortality in Childhood: Lessons from WFS', in Cleland and Hobcraft (eds.), *Reproductive Change*.

RAMANUJAM, C. (1988), 'Correlates of Infant Mortality in a Rural Area of Tamil Nadu', in Jain and Visaria (eds.), *Infant Mortality in India*.

RAO, P. S. S. and RICHARD, J. (1984), 'Socio-Economic and Demographic Correlates of Medical Care and Health Practices', *Journal of Biosocial Science*, vol. 16, no. 3.

Registrar General of India (1981*a*), *Survey of Infant and Child Mortality 1979*, New Delhi: Government of India.

—— (1981*b*), *Levels, Trends and Differentials in Fertility 1979*, New Delhi: Government of India.

—— (1983*a*), *Census of India 1981, Series 22: Uttar Pradesh, Report and Tables Based on 5 per cent Sample Data*, New Delhi: Government of India.

—— (1983*b*), *Census of India 1981, Series 20: Tamil Nadu, Report and Tables Based on 5 per cent Sample Data*, New Delhi: Government of India.

—— (1988*a*), *Female Age at Marriage: An Analysis of 1981 Census Data*, New Delhi: Government of India.

—— (1988*b*), *Birth Interval Differentials in India*, New Delhi: Government of India.

—— (1991), *Census of India 1991: Provisional Population Tables*, New Delhi: Government of India.

RINDFUSS, R. R. and MORGAN, S.P. (1983), 'Marriage, Sex and the First Birth Interval: The Quiet Revolution in Asia', *Population and Development Review*, vol. 9, no. 2.

RIZVI, N. (1983), 'Effects of Food Policy on Intrahousehold Food Distribution in Bangladesh', *Food and Nutrition Bulletin*, vol. 5, no. 4.

RODRIGUEZ, G. and CLELAND, J. (1980), 'Socio-economic Determinants of Marital Fertility in Twenty Countries: A Multivariate Analysis', in *World Fertility Survey Conference 1980: Record of Proceedings*, London: WFS.

ROSENZWEIG, M. R. and SCHULTZ, T. P. (1982), 'Child Mortality and Fertility in Colombia: Individual and Community Effects', *Health Policy and Education*, vol. 2, nos. 3–4.

RUTSTEIN, S. O. (1983), 'Infant and Child Mortality: Levels, Trends and Demographic Differentials', *WFS Comparative Studies*, no. 24.

SCHULTZ, T. P. (1982), 'Women's Work and their Status: Rural Indian Evidence of Labour Market and Environment Effects on Sex Differences in Childhood Mortality', in A. Anker, M. Buvinic, and N. H. Youssef (eds.), *Women's Role and Population Trends in the Third World*, London: Croom Helm.

SCRIMSHAW, S. (1978), 'Infant Mortality and Behaviour in the Regulation of Family Size', *Population and Development Review*, vol. 4, no. 3.

SCRIMSHAW, N. S., TAYLOR, C. E. and GORDON, J. E. (1968), *Interaction of Nutrition and Infection*, Geneva: World Health Organization.

SEN, A. K. (1987), 'Women, Well-Being and Agency', lecture presented to the seminar on Women's Issues in Development Policy, International Center for Research on Women, Washington, DC.

_____ and SENGUPTA, S. (1983), 'Malnutrition of Rural Children and the Sex Bias', *Economic and Political Weekly Annual Number*, vol. 18, nos. 19–21.

SHARMA, U. M. (1980*a*), *Women, Work and Property in North-west India*, London: Tavistock.

_____ (1980*b*), 'Purdah and Public Space', in A. de Souza (ed.), *Women in Contemporary India and South Asia*, New Delhi: Manohar Publishers.

SHÉKAR, M. (1983), *Infant Feeding Practices in an Urban Slum—A Report*, New Delhi: National Institute of Public Cooperation and Child Development.

SINGH, A. M. (1978), 'Women and the Family: Coping with Poverty in the *Bastis* of Delhi', in A. de Souza (ed.), *The Indian City: Poverty, Ecology and Urban Development*, New Delhi: Manohar Publishers.

_____ (1984), 'Rural-to-Urban Migration of Women in India: Patterns and Implications', in J.T. Fawcett, S.E. Khoo, and P.C. Smith (eds.), *Women in the Cities of Asia: Migration and Urban Adaptation*, Boulder, Colo.: Westview Press.

_____ and DE SOUZA, A. (1980), *The Urban Poor: Slum and Pavement Dwellers in the Major Cities of India*, New Delhi: Manohar Press.

SINGH, S. and CASTERLINE, J. B. (1985), 'The Socio-economic Determinants of Fertility', in Cleland and Hobcraft (eds.), *Reproductive Change*.

SINGH, S., GORDON, J. E. and WYON, J. B. (1962), 'Medical Care in Fatal Illnesses of a Rural Punjab Population: Some Social, Biological and Cultural Factors and their Ecological Implications', *Indian Journal of Medical Research*, vol. 50, no. 6.

SMITH, P. C. (1983), 'The Impact of Age at Marriage and Proportions Marrying on Fertility', in Bulatao and Lee (eds.), *Determinants of Fertility*.

SOERADJI, B. and HATMADJI, S. H. (1982), 'Contraceptive Use in Java, Bali: A Multivariate Analysis of the Determinants of Contraceptive Use', World Fertility Survey Scientific Reports, no. 24.

SOPHER, D. E. (ed.) (1980), *An Exploration of India: Geographical Perspectives on Society and Culture*, London: Longman.

SRINIVAS, M. N. (1976), *Remembered Village*, Berkeley, Calif.: University of California Press.

SUSSMAN, G. D. (1980), 'Parisian Infants and Norman Wet Nurses in the Early Nineteenth Century: A Statistical Study', in R.I. Rotberg and T. K. Rabb (eds.), *Marriage and Fertility: Studies in Interdisciplinary History*, Princeton, NJ: Princeton University Press.

THOMPSON, M., NAWAB ALI, V. and CASTERLINE, J. B. (1982), 'Collecting Demographic Data in Bangladesh: Evidence from Tape Recorded Interviews', World Fertility Survey Scientific Reports, no. 41.

TRUSSELL, J. and REINIS, K. I. (1989), 'Age at First Marriage and Age at First Birth', *Population Bulletin of the United Nations*.

TUCKER, K. and SANJUR, D. (1988), 'Maternal Employment and Child Nutrition in Panama', *Social Science and Medicine*, vol. 26.

United Nations (1961), *The Mysore Population Study*, New York: United Nations, Department of Economic and Social Affairs.

—— (1983), *Manual X: Indirect Techniques for Demographic Estimation*, New York: United Nations, Department of International Economic and Social Affairs.

—— (1985), *Socio-economic Differentials in Child Mortality in Developing Countries*, New York: United Nations, Department of International Economic and Social Affairs.

United Nations Population Division (1983), 'Recent Trends and Conditions of Fertility', paper presented at the UN Expert Group Meeting on Fertility and Family, New Delhi.

VAN DE WALLE, F. (1975), 'Migration and Fertility in Ticino', *Population Studies*, vol. 29, no. 3.

VISARIA, L. (1988), 'Sex Differentials in Nutritional Status and Survival during Infancy and Childhood', paper presented to the International Union for the Scientific Study of Population Conference on Women's Position and Demographic Change in the Course of Development, Asker, Norway.

VISARIA, P. M. (1967), 'The Sex Ratio of the Population of India and

Pakistan and Regional Variations during 1901–61', in A. Bose (ed.), *Patterns of Population Change in India 1951–61*, Bombay: Allied Publishers.

WARE, H. (1977), 'The Relationship between Infant Mortality and Fertility: Replacement and Insurance Effects', *Proceedings of the IUSSP Conference, Mexico City*, Liège, Belgium: International Union for the Scientific Study of Population.

―― (1984), 'Effects of Maternal Education, Women's Roles and Child Care on Child Mortality', *Population and Development Review*, supplement to vol. 10.

WATKINS, S. C. (1986), 'Regional Patterns of Nuptiality in Western Europe, 1870–1960', in Coale and Watkins (eds.), *The Decline of Fertility*.

WEINBERGER, M. B. and HELIGMAN, L. (1987), 'Do Social and Economic Variables Differentially Affect Male and Female Mortality?' paper presented to the 1989 Annual Meeting of the Population Association of America.

WISER, W. and WISER, C. (1971), *Behind Mud Walls 1930–1960*, Berkeley, Calif.: University of California Press.

WODEHOUSE, P. G. (1926), *The Heart of a Goof*, London: Herbert Jenkins.

WOOLF, V. (1929), *A Room of One's Own*, London: Harcourt, Brace, Jovanovich.

World Health Organization (1978), *Lay Reporting of Health Information*, Geneva: WHO.

―― (1983), *Measuring Change in Nutritional Status: Guidelines for Assessing the Nutritional Impact of Supplementary Feeding Programmes for Vulnerable Groups*, Geneva: WHO.

―― (1986), *Health Implications of Sex Discrimination in Childhood*, Geneva: WHO.

WRIGLEY, E. A. (1969), *Population and History*, London: World University Press.

WYATT, H. V. (1984), 'The Popularity of Injections in the Third World: Origins and Consequences for Poliomyelitis', *Social Science and Medicine*, vol. 19, no. 2.

―― WYON, J. B. and GORDON, J. E. (1971), *The Khanna Study*, Cambridge, Mass.: Harvard University Press.

―― HEER, D. M., PARTHASARATHY, N R., and GORDON, J. E. (1966), 'Delayed Marriage and Prospects for Fewer Births in Punjab Villages', *Demography*, vol. 3, no. 2.

YAUKEY, D., ROBERTS, B. J. and GRIFFITHS, W. (1965), 'Husbands' and Wives' Responses to a Fertility Survey', *Population Studies*, vol. 19, no. 1.

Index